OXFORD MEDICAL PUBLICATIONS

Cardiovascular
Imaging

T0177522

Oxford Specialist Handbooks published and forthcoming

General Oxford Specialist Handbooks
A Resuscitation Room Guide
Addiction Medicine
Perioperative Medicine,
Second Edition
Post-Operative Complications,
Second edition

Oxford Specialist Handbooks in Anaesthesia
Cardiac Anaesthesia
General Thoracic Anaesthesia
Neuroanaesthesia
Obstetric Anaesthesia
Paediatric Anaesthesia
Regional Anaesthesia, Stimulation
and Ultrasound Techniques

Oxford Specialist Handbooks in Cardiology
Adult Congenital Heart Disease
Cardiac Catheterization and
Coronary Intervention
Cardiovascular Imaging
Echocardiography
Fetal Cardiology
Heart Disease in Pregnancy
Heart Failure
Hypertension
Inherited Cardiac Disease
Nuclear Cardiology
Pacemakers and ICDs

Oxford Specialist Handbooks in Critical Care
Advanced Respiratory Critical Care

Oxford Specialist Handbooks in End of Life Care
End of Life Care in Cardiology
End of Life Care in Dementia
End of Life Care in Nephrology
End of Life Care in Respiratory
Disease
End of Life Care in the Intensive
Care Unit

Oxford Specialist Handbooks in Neurology
Epilepsy
Parkinson's Disease and Other
Movement Disorders
Stroke Medicine

Oxford Specialist Handbooks in Paediatrics
Paediatric Endocrinology
and Diabetes
Paediatric Dermatology
Paediatric Gastroenterology,
Hepatology, and Nutrition
Paediatric Haematology and
Oncology
Paediatric Nephrology
Paediatric Neurology
Paediatric Radiology
Paediatric Respiratory Medicine

Oxford Specialist Handbooks in Psychiatry
Child and Adolescent Psychiatry
Old Age Psychiatry

Oxford Specialist Handbooks in Radiology
Interventional Radiology
Musculoskeletal Imaging

Oxford Specialist Handbooks in Surgery
Cardiothoracic Surgery
Hand Surgery
Hepato-pancreatobiliary Surgery
Oral Maxillo Facial Surgery
Neurosurgery
Operative Surgery, Second Edition
Otolaryngology and Head and Neck
Surgery
Plastic and Reconstructive Surgery
Surgical Oncology
Urological Surgery
Vascular Surgery

Oxford Specialist Handbooks in Cardiology
Cardiovascular Imaging

Edited by

Paul Leeson

Consultant Cardiologist
John Radcliffe Hospital and
BHF Fellow, University of Oxford
Oxford, UK

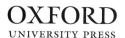

OXFORD
UNIVERSITY PRESS

OXFORD

UNIVERSITY PRESS

Great Clarendon Street, Oxford OX2 6DP

Oxford University Press is a department of the University of Oxford.
It furthers the University's objective of excellence in research, scholarship,
and education by publishing worldwide in

Oxford New York

Auckland Cape Town Dar es Salaam Hong Kong Karachi
Kuala Lumpur Madrid Melbourne Mexico City Nairobi
New Delhi Shanghai Taipei Toronto

With offices in

Argentina Austria Brazil Chile Czech Republic France Greece
Guatemala Hungary Italy Japan Poland Portugal Singapore
South Korea Switzerland Thailand Turkey Ukraine Vietnam

Oxford is a registered trade mark of Oxford University Press
in the UK and in certain other countries

Published in the United States
by Oxford University Press Inc., New York

British Library Cataloguing in Publication Data
Data available

Library of Congress Control Number: 2011925400

Typeset by Glyph International, Bangalore, India
Printed in Great Britain on acid-free paper by
Ashford Colour Press Ltd, Gosport, Hampshire

ISBN 978–0–19–956845–1

10 9 8 7 6 5 4 3 2 1

v

Foreword

During the last 20 years we have seen an unimaginable progress in imaging techniques for cardiovascular disease. However, this progress came with the need for specialization. In the old days a cardiologist could be trained in the few imaging techniques available and was able to apply them. Now, even cardiologists specializing in imaging often only choose one or two imaging methods in order to be able to acquire all the expertise necessary and maintain the skills in daily practice.

Appropriate use of the imaging techniques depend on the referrals to the imaging tests. These referrals come from cardiologists, but more often from other specialists e.g. internists, neurologists, and general practitioners. During their training in medical school, and as a postgraduate, these physicians have often been taught about the different imaging techniques separately and it can be difficult to keep up to speed with the developing technologies. Therefore inappropriate referrals for specific cardiac tests can occur and attribute to the financial burden in health care.

There have been books on cardiovascular imaging, but most of them have been too extensive and are unlikely to be read by those who refer patients for imaging tests. Paul Leeson has succeeded in editing a short but comprehensive manual which can be managed by all who are willing to achieve the best for their patients. Using the very successful format of the Oxford Specialist Handbook series, *Cardiovascular Imaging* provides an excellent overview of the current technology in X-Ray, echocardiography, cardiac magnetic resonance imaging, angiography, nuclear imaging, and computed tomography. The reader finds the indications, results and pitfalls of the different methods. All this is easily readable and focuses on the clinically relevant issues. I am convinced that this concept will fly and help to increase the appropriate use of cardiac imaging.

Harald Becher MD PhD FRCP
Professor of Medicine
Heart & Stroke Foundation Chair for Cardiovascular Research
Mazankowski Alberta Heart Institute,
University of Alberta Hospital
Edmonton, Canada
24th February 2011

Preface

'An accurate drawing, accompanied by a few words to the point, often conveys more than several paragraphs of text'. This idea is evident throughout the modality-based cardiovascular imaging books within the Oxford Specialist Handbook series. These handbooks provide practical, hands on advice for people who are performing imaging everyday and need to know how to collect good quality images and interpret the findings.

Cardiovascular Imaging now applies this idea to address the world of cardiovascular imaging from a multi-modality perspective. The book was written to be useful to two types of people. The first are those early in cardiology or radiology training, whether or not they have a particular interest in cardiovascular imaging, who want to get to grips with the whole range of imaging techniques available. The book should help these people understand how the images are generated and how you can begin to interpret and use the images produced. For those who go on to specialize in cardiovascular imaging this information can be used as the background, and springboard, to more specialized texts. The second group of people are all those who may never themselves be involved with acquisition of cardiovascular imaging data but want to understand the range of modalities and how best to apply - or request - the techniques to look at different pathologies.

The world of cardiovascular imaging is fast moving and new techniques are developing alongside application of existing modalities to different pathologies. The environment benefits from the in-depth knowledge specialists develop in individual modalities, or even specific techniques, or applications, within the same modality! Multi-modality texts based on core, fundamental principles offer the common ground from which you can develop personal expertise in cardiovascular imaging.

PL
February 2011

Acknowledgements

I am grateful to all my junior and senior colleagues who I work with in cardiology. Their contributions, whether in discussions, when reviewing cases or directly through writing chapters, made this book possible.

Contents

Detailed contents   *xiii*
Contributors   *xvii*
List of abbreviations   *xix*
Further reading   *xxiii*

Image acquisition: modalities and views

1 **Imaging modalities**   *1*
2 **Imaging planes**   *63*

Applied imaging: anatomy, function, and pathology

3 **Left ventricular function**   *97*
4 **Myocardium**   *125*
5 **Coronary artery disease**   *137*
6 **Right ventricle**   *153*
7 **Valves**   *169*
8 **Pericardium**   *209*
9 **Aorta**   *243*
10 **Congenital heart disease**   *259*
11 **Arrhythmias**   *285*

Index   *301*

Detailed contents

Contributors *xvii*

List of abbreviations *xix*

Further reading *xxiii*

1 Imaging modalities 1

Cardiovascular imaging *2*
Chest X-ray *4*
Coronary angiography *6*
Left ventriculography and aortography *10*
Percutaneous coronary intervention *10*
Intravascular ultrasound *12*
Optical coherence tomography *14*
Transthoracic echocardiography *16*
Transoesophageal echocardiography *28*
Three-dimensional echocardiography *32*
Intracardiac ultrasound *32*
Cardiovascular magnetic resonance *34*
Cardiac computed tomography *40*
CT coronary angiography *46*
Coronary calcium scoring *48*
Myocardial perfusion scintigraphy *50*
Radionuclide ventriculography (RNV) *60*
Positron emission tomography (PET) *62*

2 Imaging planes 63

Imaging planes *64*
Long axis: four-chamber view *66*
Long axis: five-chamber view *68*
Long axis: two-chamber view (LV) *70*
Long axis: two-chamber view (RV) *72*
Long axis: three-chamber view *74*
Short axis: aortic valve view *76*
Short axis: mitral valve view *78*
Short axis: left ventricular view *80*
Right ventricular inflow view *82*
Right ventricular outflow view *84*
Inferior vena cava views *86*
Aortic views *88*
Pulmonary vein views *90*
Coronary sinus views *90*
Polar view *92*
3D reconstructions *94*

3 Left ventricular function 97

Left ventricle 98
Left ventricular function 100
Chest X-ray 104
Echocardiography 106
Cardiac magnetic resonance 112
Radionuclide ventriculography (RNV) 114
Single-photon emission computed tomography (SPECT) 116
Positron emission tomography (PET) 118
Cardiac CT 120
Angiography 122

4 Myocardium 125

Myocardial imaging 126
Echocardiography 128
Cardiac magnetic resonance 132
Cardiac CT 136
Coronary angiography 136

5 Coronary artery disease 137

Coronary artery disease 138
Myocardial ischaemia 140
Coronary angiography 144
Cardiac CT 146
Cardiac magnetic resonance 148
Nuclear cardiology 150
Echocardiography 152

6 Right ventricle 153

Right ventricle 154
Right ventricular structure and function 156
Echocardiography 158
Cardiac magnetic resonance 162
Radionuclide imaging 164
Cardiac catheterization 166

7 Valves 169

Valves 170
Valve structure 172
Valve function 176
Valve masses 180
Severity assessment 184
Prosthetic valve function 186
Mitral stenosis 188
Mitral regurgitation 192
Aortic stenosis 194
Aortic regurgitation 198
Tricuspid valve 200

Pulmonary valve *202*
Prosthetic valves *204*

8 Pericardium *209*

Pericardium *210*
Chest X-ray *212*
Echocardiography *214*
Cardiac CT *216*
Cardiac magnetic resonance *218*
Coronary angiography *220*
Nuclear cardiology *220*
Acute pericarditis *222*
Constrictive pericarditis *224*
Pericardial effusion and tamponade *228*
Pericardial tumours *234*
Congenital pericardial disorders *236*
Pericardiocentesis *240*
Pericardiotomy *240*

9 Aorta *243*

Aortic atherosclerosis *244*
Aortic aneurysm *246*
Aortic dissection *248*
Intramural haematoma *252*
Marfan syndrome *254*
Aortic coarctation *256*

10 Congenital heart disease *259*

Congenital heart disease *260*
Chest X-ray *262*
Echocardiography *264*
Transoesophageal echocardiography *266*
Cardiac magnetic resonance *268*
Cardiac CT *270*
Cardiac catheterization *272*
Atrial and ventricular septal defects *274*
Aortic coarctation *276*
Transposition of the great arteries *278*
Tetralogy of Fallot *280*
Aberrant coronary anatomy *282*
Patent ductus arteriosus *282*
Major aorto-pulmonary collateral arteries (MAPCAs) *282*
Pulmonary arterial hypertension including Eisenmenger's
    syndrome *284*

11 Arrhythmias *285*

Arrhythmias *286*
Atrial arrhythmias *288*
Supraventricular tachycardia *290*

Ventricular tachycardia 292
Ventricular fibrillation 294
Cardiac arrest 294
Arrhythmogenic right ventricular cardiomyopathy (ARVC) 294
Catheter ablation of arrhythmias 296

Index 301

Contributors

Sincere thanks are due to the following people (in alphabetical order) for their expert contributions which formed the following sections.

David Adlam
Specialist Registrar in Cardiology,
John Radcliffe Hospital,
Oxford, UK
Coronary angiography

Harald Becher
Professor of Cardiology,
Mazankowski Alberta Heart
Institute, Edmonton, Canada
Myocardium

Lucy Hudsmith
Consultant Cardiologist,
University Hospitals NHS Trust,
Birmingham, UK
Congenital heart disease

Merzaka Lazdam
Clinical Research Fellow,
John Radcliffe Hospital,
Oxford, UK
Imaging planes

Andrew Mitchell
Consultant Cardiologist, Jersey
General Hospital, St Helier,
Jersey, UK
Aorta, arrhythmias

Jim Newton
Consultant Cardiologist,
John Radcliffe Hospital,
Oxford, UK
Valvular imaging

Edward Nicol
Consultant Cardiologist,
Royal Brompton Hospital,
London, UK
Cardiac CT

Kal Asress
Clinical Research Fellow and
Specialist Registrar in Cardiology,
Cardiovascular Division,
The Rayne Institute,
St Thomas Hospital,
London, UK
Aorta, arrhythmias

Nik Sabharwal
Consultant Cardiologist, John
Radcliffe Hospital, Oxford, UK
Nuclear cardiology

Cezary Szmigielski
Department of Internal Medicine,
Medical University of Warsaw,
Warsaw, Poland
Myocardium, left and right ventricles

All other sections were written by Paul Leeson

List of abbreviations

2D	two-dimensional
3D	three-dimensional
AF	atrial fibrillation
AP	accessory pathway
AR	aortic regurgitation
AS	aortic stenosis
ASD	atrial septal defect
ASE	Agatston score equivalent, ASE American Society of Echocardiography
AV	atrioventricular
AVNRT	atrioventricular nodal re-entry tachycardia
AVRT	atrioventricular re-entry tachycardia
CABG	coronary artery bypass graft
CFM	colour flow mapping
CMR	cardiac magnetic resonance
CO	cardiac output
CT	computed tomography
CTA	CT coronary angiography
CW	continuous wave
DET	deceleration time
EBCT	electron beam computed tomography
EDV	end-diastolic volume
EF	ejection fraction
HASTE	half-Fourier acquisition single-shot turbo spin echo
HLA	horizontal long axis
ICD	implantable cardioverter defibrillator
ICE	intracardiac echocardiography
IVC	inferior vena cava
IVRT	isovolumetric relaxation time
IVUS	intravascular ultrasound
LA	left atrium
LAO	left anterior oblique
LGE	late gadolinium enhancement
LLPV	left lower pulmonary vein
LUPV	left upper pulmonary vein

LV	left ventricle
LVEF	left ventricular ejection fraction
LVID	left ventricular internal diameter
LVOT	left ventricular outflow tract
LVPW	left ventricular posterior wall
LVS	left ventricular septum
MDCT	multi-detector computed tomography
MI	myocardial infarction
MR	magnetic resonance, mitral regurgitation
MS	mitral stenosis
MV	mitral valve
MVA	mitral valve area
NSTEMI	non-ST-elevation myocardial infarction
OCT	optical coherence tomography
PA	pulmonary artery
PCI	percutaneous coronary intervention
PDA	patent ductus arteriosus
PET	positron emission tomography
PFO	patent foramen ovale
PHT	pressure half time
P_{max}	peak pressure
P_{mean}	mean pressure
PR	pulmonary regurgitation
PS	pulmonary stenosis
PV	pulmonary valve
PW	pulsed wave
RA	right atrium
RAO	right anterior oblique
RLPV	right lower pulmonary vein
RNV	radionuclide ventriculography
RUPV	right upper pulmonary vein
RV	right ventricle
RVEF	right ventricular ejection fraction
RVOT	right ventricular outflow tract
RWMA	regional wall motion abnormality
SPECT	single-photon emission computed tomography
SSFP	steady state free precession
STEMI	ST-elevation myocardial infarction
SV	stroke volume
SVC	superior vena cava

TAPSE	tricuspid annular plane systolic excursion
TDI	tissue Doppler imaging
TGA	transposition of the great arteries
TOE	transoesophageal echocardiography
TR	tricuspid regurgitation
TV	tricuspid valve
VLA	vertical long axis
V_{max}	peak velocity
V_{mean}	mean velocity
VSD	ventricular septal defect
VT	ventricular tachycardia
VTI	velocity–time integral
WMSI	wall motion score index
WPW	Wolff–Parkinson–White

Further reading

Textbooks (in alphabetical order)

Leeson, P., Mitchell, A.R.J., and Becher, H. (eds) (2007). *Echocardiography*. Oxford University Press, Oxford.

Myerson, S.G., Francis, J., and Neubauer, S. (eds) (2010). *Cardiovascular Magnetic Resonance*. Oxford University Press, Oxford.

Nicol, E., Stirrup, J., Kelion, A.D., Padley, S.P.G. *et al. Cardiovascular Computed Tomography*. Oxford University Press, Oxford. (In press).

Sabharwal, N., Chee Yee-Loong, and Kelion, A. (2008). *Nuclear Cardiology*. Oxford University Press, Oxford.

St John Sutton, M. Leppo, J. (2004). *Clinical Cardiovascular Imaging: A Companion to Braunwald's Heart Disease*. W.B. Saunders, Philadelphia, PA.

Zamorano, J.L., Bax, J.J., Rademakers, F.E., Knuuti, J. (eds) (2010). *The ESC Textbook of Cardiovascular Imaging*. Springer, London.

Websites

American Heart Association http://www.americanheart.org/

American Society of Echocardiography http://www.asecho.org

British Cardiovascular Society http://www.bcs.com/

British Heart Foundation http://www.bhf.org.uk/

British Nuclear Cardiology Society http://www.bncs.org.uk

British Society of Cardiovascular Imaging http://www.bsci.org.uk

British Society of Cardiovascular Magnetic Resonance http://www.bscmr.org

British Society of Echocardiography http://www.bsecho.org

European Association of Echocardiography http://www.escardio.org/bodies/associations/EAE

European Society of Cardiology http://www.escardio.org/

European Working Group for Cardiovascular Magnetic Resonance http://www.escardio.org/communities/working-groups/eurocmr

European Working Group for Nuclear Cardiology and Cardiac CT http://www.escardio.org/communities/working-groups/nuclear-cardiology/pages/welcome.aspx

Society for Cardiovascular Magnetic Resonance http://www.scmr.org

Chapter 1

Imaging modalities

Cardiovascular imaging *2*
Chest X-ray *4*
Coronary angiography *6*
Left ventriculography and aortography *10*
Percutaneous coronary intervention *10*
Intravascular ultrasound *12*
Optical coherence tomography *14*
Transthoracic echocardiography *16*
Transoesophageal echocardiography *28*
Three-dimensional echocardiography *32*
Intracardiac ultrasound *32*
Cardiovascular magnetic resonance *34*
Cardiac computed tomography *40*
CT coronary angiography *46*
Coronary calcium scoring *48*
Myocardial perfusion scintigraphy *50*
Radionuclide ventriculography (RNV) *60*
Positron emission tomography (PET) *62*

Cardiovascular imaging

Imaging is of paramount importance in assessment of cardiovascular disease. The diagnosis of disease has been revolutionized by the ability to gain high-resolution imaging of all aspects of the heart and vessels, and we are now able to visualize and assess function of everything 'from the heart to the capillary'. As a result multiple modalities and approaches are used and the area has matured to a stage where it is not possible for everyone—or anyone—to have the same high level of specialist knowledge across all modalities. For the newcomer the range of options can appear confusing. Fortunately, some common approaches to cardiovascular imaging have developed that are transferable across modalities and allow anyone to pick up an image and begin to interpret what is seen. The basic things to get to grips with are the follwoing.

- Imaging planes—there is a recognizable series of imaging planes of the heart that allows anyone to orientate themselves to a particular structure based on some clues from the image.
- Diseases tend to relate to structures and areas—disease processes tend to affect a predominant area of the heart (although abnormalities in one area may affect other aspects). Different modalities are better at studying different aspects. In general:
  - myocardium—MR/SPECT/PET
  - cardiac function—Echo/CMR
  - valve structure and function—echo
  - coronaries—angiography/CT
  - central vessels—MR/CT
  - peripheral vessels—CT/MR/ultrasound.
- Advantages of particular modalities relate to the patient and the disease:
  - Echo—acute settings, high volume, real time
  - MR—unlimited by body habitus, any image plane
  - CT—rapid collection of volume dataset.
- Disadvantages of modalities relate to how the images are acquired:
  - Echo—range limited by penetration of ultrasound
  - MR—limited by need for magnetic field, having receivers close to the patient, acquisition over several cardiac cycles
  - CT—limited by need for radiation
  - SPECT—limited by resolution and need for radiation.
- Availability and users—Use of modalities in different centres is best determined by available resources and local expertise. The value of any modality chosen to investigate the patient is nearly always determined by the individuals involved in the data collection:
  - the ability of the physician to make the right differential diagnoses
  - the ability of the operator to acquire the appropriate best-quality images
  - the expertise of the individual who interprets the image.

Chest X-ray

Background
- The chest X-ray remains the most universal and simplest cardiac imaging investigation.

Advantages
- Wide availability in acute and non-acute setting in hospital.
- Provides information on structures outside the heart to aid differential diagnosis.
- Basis of more advanced techniques such as CT and angiography.

Disadvantages
- Use of radiation.
- 2D.
- Compression of information from the whole of the patient's chest into a single plane with resultant loss of information.

Pathology on chest X-ray
The key findings identified on chest X-ray that may prompt further cardiovascular imaging are:
- Changes in heart shape or size—these may be due to changes in the myocardium (hypertrophy), chamber size (left atrial enlargement, left ventricular failure) or pericardial (pericardial effusion).
- Changes in lung fields—features of fluid, either interstitial or pleural, suspicious for left ventricular failure.
- Changes in aortic shadow—aortic aneurysm, dissection.
- Changes in tissue—calcification over the heart shadow (e.g. pericardial disease or valvular calcification).

Basics of chest X-ray
The standard chest X-ray for cardiology investigation is based on the PA (postero-anterior) projection (Fig. 1.1), but in acute settings, with patients in bed, it may be recorded in AP (antero-posterior) format. Lateral views are not often additionally required unless further information on the lung lobes or position of pacing leads is considered necessary. Following the initial chest X-ray, the usual next step is likely to be a further imaging modality.

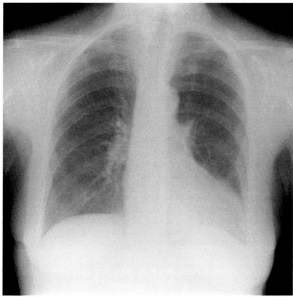

Fig. 1.1 Chest X-ray in standard PA projection allows study of cardiac size and silhouette as well as lungs, diaphragm, and skeletal structures in the chest.

Coronary angiography

Background

Coronary angiography is one of the first cardiovascular imaging techniques learnt during training in cardiology and is the one most closely linked to cardiology practice and sub-specialization. It is one of the oldest techniques in cardiology. The technique involves injection of radio-opaque contrast via a catheter placed in the coronary ostia (Fig. 1.2) accompanied by simultaneous fluoroscopy to provide a real-time image of coronary luminal anatomy.

Pathology and coronary angiography

Coronary angiography is excellent for studying the coronary lumen. It provides information on:

- Coronary luminal narrowing, usually caused by atherosclerosis in the vessel wall, in order to identify the number and severity of coronary stenoses that may impair distal perfusion, causing symptomatic angina.
- Rupture of coronary atheromatous plaques, central to the patho-physiology of acute coronary syndromes and myocardial infarction with possible associated presence of thrombus.
- Some indication of coronary flow through speed of filling of artery and distal microvascular appearances.
- Further potential diagnostic information central to the processs of percutaneous coronary intervention (PCI) such as anomalous coronary anatomy or dissection.

The other imaging techniques available during the coronary angiography procedure are ventriculography and aortic assessment (p 10).

- Ventriculography allows assessment of left ventricular function including regional wall motion abnormalities (when this information is not available from other imaging modalities or a second assessment is required) and severity of mitral regurgitation (based on a qualitative assessment of the amount of contrast that passes back into the left atrium). Aortic root dimensions are also demonstrated.
- Aortography is indicated for more precise assessment of the dimensions of the aortic root (particularly important in the surgical workup of aortic valve disease) and severity of aortic regurgitation (based on a qualitative assessment of the amount of contrast that passes back into the left ventricle) Aortography can also be used to identify the origin of coronary vessels or grafts.

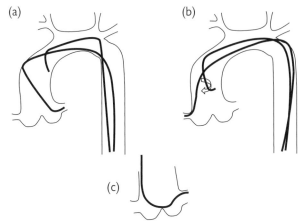

Fig. 1.2 Positioning and shape of catheters within the aortic root. (a) The Judkins left 4 catheter is shaped to enter the left coronary ostium. (b) The Judkins right coronary catheter requires careful clockwise rotation prior to engagement of the right coronary ostium. (c) The Amplatzer catheter is shaped differently and sits across the aortic root.

Basics of coronary angiography

The team

The specialist team needed to acquire coronary angiographic data comprises an operator, a scrub nurse or assistant, a runner nurse, a cardiac physiologist, and a radiographer. The patient is continuously monitored by ECG and oxygen saturations in addition to the continuous measurement of pressure transduced from the catheter. Patients are not usually anaesthetized, which allows assessment of symptoms during the procedure, but sedation may be used.

Vascular access

Percutaneous arterial puncture is usually performed by the Seldinger technique. The most common routes of access are via the femoral or radial arteries. Occasionally, a brachial cut-down may be used when other routes of access are difficult, in which case an arteriotomy under direct vision rather than a percutaneous approach is used. Haemostasis at the end of the procedure may be achieved with manual pressure or an external compression device (such as a Femstop for femoral procedures or a TR band for radial procedures). There are a number of arterial sealing devices for femoral punctures (e.g. Angioseal® and Starclosure® devices). Once a sheath (usually 5–8 French depending on the nature of the planned procedure and the route of access) is sited in the artery, a catheter is passed over a guidewire to the aortic route. After removal of the guidewire the coronary ostia can be engaged by careful advancement and manipulation of the catheter.

Coronary catheters

The catheters used for coronary angiography and percutaneous intervention are variously shaped to facilitate engagement of the coronary otium and also to provide good back-up support to prevent the catheter backing out of the coronary ostium when angioplasty wires, balloons, and stents are advanced into the coronary artery during PCI.

Fluoroscopic projections

Coronary angiography provides a 2D image of what is in reality a 3D structure (i.e. the lumen of the coronary arteries as they pass around the epicardial surface of the heart). Therefore views from multiple angles are used to overcome problems of vessel overlap and foreshortening. These projections should be individually tailored to each patient's anatomy and the area of clinical interest, and are adapted from a number of standard projections (Fig. 1.3). Further detailed images on projections can be found in Mitchell A (2008) et al. See further reading p. xix.

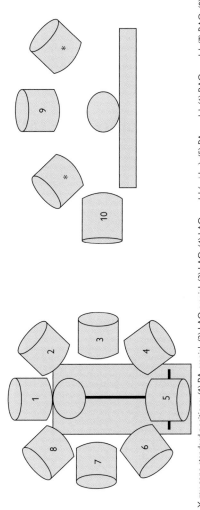

Fig. 1.3 X-ray cone standard positions: (1) PA cranial, (2) LAO cranial, (3) LAO, (4) LAO caudal (spider), (5) PA caudal, (6) RAO caudal, (7) RAO, (8) RAO cranial. These views are taken at an angle to the horizontal (*) with the exception of PA (9), which is taken vertically, and lateral (10), which is taken from the patient's side.

Left ventriculography and aortography

By placing a catheter in the left ventricle, injecting contrast, and then performing fluoroscopy, images in multiple planes of the left ventricular cavity
can be generated (Fig. 1.4). These views can also provide a rough guide to
mitral valve disease. The extent of calcification can be assessed and regurgitation quantified based on the amount of contrast that passes across the
mitral valve during systole.

By placing the pigtail catheter in the aorta, injecting and recording fluros-
copy images of the lumen of the aorta can be obtained (Fig. 1.5). This can
be useful for assessment of aortic dissection or aneurysm.

Percutaneous coronary intervention

In addition to diagnostic information on the location and severity of coronary disease, coronary angiography is used to guide percutaneous intervention. Angioplasty is based on the same Seldinger principles as angiography. A fine angioplasty guidewire is passed from a guide catheter placed
in the coronary ostium and used to cross the target lesion. Angioplasty
balloons and subsequently stents can be guided into position along this
wire. Fluoroscopy is used for direct visualization of angioplasty wires, balloons, stents, etc., thus allowing the operator to manipulate them into the
desired position. Simultaneous angiography is used to delineate the target
lesion during this process and to observe the effects of balloon inflation
and/or subsequent stent deployment on the target stenosis and the coronary
artery as a whole.

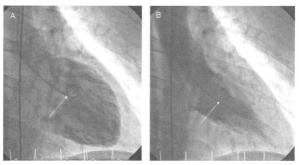

Fig. 1.4 Left ventriculogram in (A) diastole and (B) systole taken in the RAO projection. A pigtail catheter (arrowed) is placed in the LV cavity and during acquisition 35mL contrast is injected at 15mL/s via an automated injector.

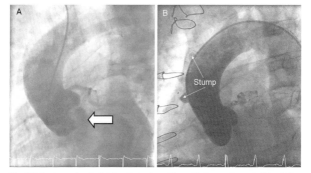

Fig. 1.5 Aortography. A pigtail catheter is positioned in the aortic root: (A) radial approach; (B) femoral approach. During acquisition in the LAO projection 40mL of contrast is injected at 20mL/s using an automated injector. (A) Significant aortic regurgitation (arrowed) into the left ventricular cavity. (B) Sternal wires following previous coronary bypass grafting and the stumps of two occluded saphenous vein grafts (arrowed) are demonstrated.

Intravascular ultrasound

Background

Intravascular ultrasound (IVUS) catheters consist of an integral ultrasound probe mounted on a flexible monorail tube which can be guided along an angioplasty wire into the coronary position of interest. Ultrasound frequencies of 10–45MHz are emitted and the reflected signal is received and transmitted to an appropriate computer for analysis and image generation. A real-time image with a frame rate of around 30 frames/s is generated. Blood appears echo-lucent, so the vessel lumen appears black whilst the soft tissue features of the vessel wall are variably echo-opaque with areas of calcification reflecting most ultrasound (therefore these appear the brightest white with an area of echo drop-out beyond). The IVUS probe can be mechanically pulled back along the angioplasty wire at a preset speed (0.5m/s) allowing images along a known length of coronary artery to be obtained and the distances separating particular features to be measured.

Pathology and IVUS

IVUS *per se* has not been shown to alter clinical endpoints in percutaneous intervention. However, it is useful as a clinical and research tool. In clinical practice the 3D assessment of coronary anatomy provided by IVUS can improve assessment of eccentric atheromatous plaque where angiographic appearances are equivocal or even misleading (Fig. 1.6). It can enhance assessment of complex lesions such as left mainstem lesions, bifurcation points, and calcific coronary disease (where concentric calcification may hinder conventional balloon inflation and rotational atherectomy may be preferred). IVUS enables a number of measures to be made to guide PCI, e.g. relative luminal diameter, and hence severity of stenosis, or internal elastic lamina of pre-stenotic, post-stenotic, and stenotic segments to estimate the original vessel diameter. These can be used to aid selection of optimal stent diameter. Measurement of lesion length during pullback can be used to select the best stent length. Following stent deployment, IVUS can be used to image stent apposition and identify areas of underdeployment. It also allows assessment of the effects of stent deployment on significant side branches which may be affected by both stent struts and plaque shift.

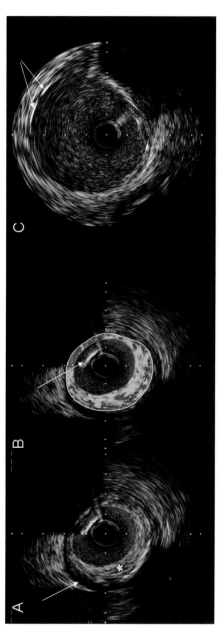

Fig. 1.6 IVUS images. (A) intracoronary image showing elliptical plaque (asterisk) around a 3mm lumen. The boundary of the external elastic lamina is clearly demarcated (arrow). (B) Post hoc image analysis can be used to estimate the plaque composition (green, fibrotic; yellow, lipid; pink, necrotic; blue, calcification). In this example the plaque is predominantly fibrotic. Note that the area of acoustic shadow cast by the angioplasty guidewire (arrow) in the top right sector leads to a misallocation of the plaque constituents in this area as being of lower echo density (i.e necrotic). (C) Image taken following stent deployment. Stent struts are seen as bright echodense points or lines (arrow).

Optical coherence tomography

Background

Like IVUS, optical coherence tomography (OCT) provides a cross-sectional assessment of the coronary lumen and part of the vessel wall (Fig. 1.7). In the case of OCT the imaging modality used is reflected light. This provides a much higher resolution (10–20µm) image of the vessel wall than IVUS but with more limited penetration. In practical terms the OCT probe is integral to a wire which can be passed via a guide catheter into the coronary position of interest. Because red blood cells scatter light, prior to OCT imaging blood must be displaced by an optically clear medium such as an appropriate contrast or crystalloid. To image longer segments of coronary artery a proximal occlusion balloon may be inflated prior to blood dispacement and an automated pullback activated at ~1mm/s with a frame rate of ~15/s.

Pathology and OCT

Currently, OCT is predominantly a research tool. The high-resolution images provided allow assessment of luminal features such as thrombus, ruptured plaque, and coronary dissection. As with IVUS, the luminal diameter and length of stenotic segment can be easily measured. However, unlike IVUS, image penetration often does not allow visualization of the internal elastic lamina and therefore estimation of the original vessel diameter. OCT provides detailed images of the location and apposition of stent struts. It is also being used experimentally to assess the duration of luminal exposure of stent struts prior to re-endothelialization and neo-intima formation following PCI. Prolonged strut exposure may be a marker of the risk for in-stent thrombosis. Despite the amazing image quality provided by OCT, a precise clinical role for this imaging modality remains to be elucidated.

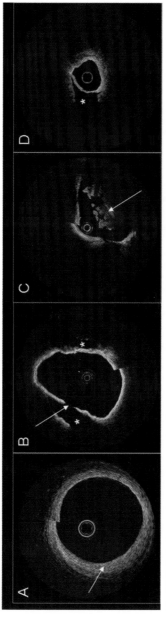

Fig. 1.7 Optical coherence tomography: examples of coronary cross-sectional images. (A) Saphenous vein graft showing concentric fibrous neo-intima (arrow). B. Subendothelial lipid-rich plaque (asterisks) with evidence of plaque rupture (arrow). (C) Intracoronary thrombus (arrow) in acute coronary syndrome. (D) Coronary dissection. The imaging wire is in the true lumen with the false lumen indicated by the asterisk.

Transthoracic echocardiography

Background
Echocardiography remains the most important diagnostic imaging tool in clinical cardiology practice. Since its development by Edler and Herz almost five decades ago, and routine clinical implementation a decade later, echocardiography has developed into an intuitive, comprehensible, and practical method for evaluating cardiac morphology and function rapidly and repeatedly.

Pathology and echocardiography
Echocardiography provides a rapid real-time assessment of cardiac anatomy and function (Fig. 1.8). It is indicated as a first-line test in virtually all types of cardiac pathology and can be used to guide any further imaging that is required.[1]

Basics of echocardiography
Ultrasound physics
- All forms of ultrasonic imaging are based on generation of high-frequency (>1MHz) acoustic pressure waves from a transducer consisting of one or more piezoelectric crystals.
- As current is passed across the crystals they deform and generate the ultrasound wave.
- The piezoelectric element also serves as a receiver. Waves returning from objects (e.g. walls, valves) deform the crystals which, in turn, generate a current that can be recorded.
- Because the velocity of sound is constant, object location (spatial resolution) can be determined based on the time it takes for a wave to return.
- The *amplitude* of the returning signal depends on the angle of incidence (surfaces perpendicular to the ultrasound beam are stronger reflectors) and the interface of acoustic impedances (greater differences such as occurs in the left ventricle at the tissue–blood interface lead to greater reflectivity).

1 Leeson, P., Mitchell, A.R.J., and Becher, H. (eds) (2007) *Echocardiography*. Oxford University Press, Oxford.

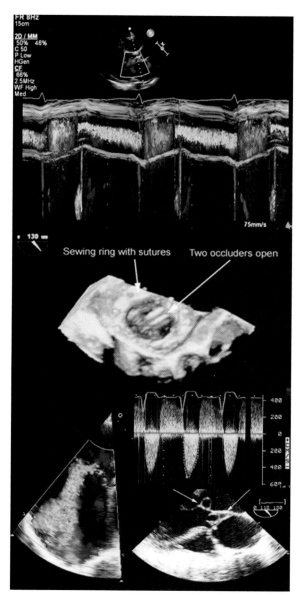

Fig. 1.8 Figure shows colour M-mode echocardiography (top), live 3D echocardiography (middle) and Doppler echocardiography (bottom).

Types of image (Fig. 1.7)

A, B, and M modes

The progress of echocardiography has followed the transition from initial images which only provided information on the *amplitude* of the returning ultrasound signal (A mode) in a single 'scan line', to representation of the amplitude as *brightness* (B mode). The next available image was the M or *motion* mode. This depicted the single scan line but represented it over *time*. The information has a high temporal resolution (>1kHz) and can study rapidly moving structures, but is still limited to single 'scan line'.

2D imaging

The main echocardiography mode used today is 2D imaging. When the ultrasound beam is swept across a chosen cardiac window, rapid sequential sampling can be performed, leading to display of multiple 'scan lines' of information and a sector image created nearly instantaneously.

3D imaging

The natural advance of echocardiography was to sweep the 'scan plane' in the axis perpendicular to the 2D image and thereby generate the data to reconstruct a 3D images. Such imaging is now also a routine function.

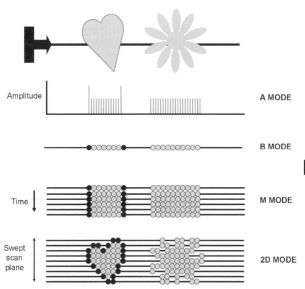

Fig. 1.9 Types of image. The A (amplitude) mode traces the amplitude of a reflection against distance from the probe (of historical interest as one of the first types of ultrasound image). The B (brightness) mode represents amplitude as intensity or brightness of a dot. The M (motion) mode traces changes in brightness over time. 2D images are generated by sweeping across the field of interest.

Doppler imaging
A powerful aspect of echocardiography is the ability to assess the speed of movement of objects with the same equipment that generates 2D and 3D structural images. Quantification of object motion is possible with Doppler-based technologies. The principles of Doppler are as follows.
- Frequencies of returning ultrasound are shifted upwards or downwards by cells depending on whether the cells are travelling towards or away from the transducer, respectively. The amount that the frequency shifts is proportional to the *velocity* of the object.
- The signal *intensity* depends on the number of cells moving at a particular velocity.
- Velocity information is depicted as a spectral pattern over time similar to the M mode (continuous and pulsed wave Doppler) or mapped to pixels as colour overlying the 2D or 3D image (colour flow imaging) (Fig. 1.10).
- The ultrasound beam must be as parallel as possible to the target for accurate measures. Off-axis angulation by >30° leads to significant underestimation of velocities.

Pulsed wave Doppler
Pulsed wave (PW) Doppler permits accurate sampling of blood velocities averaged within a limited region of interest or 'sample volume'.
- Transducer elements serve as both transmitters and receivers, permitting selective sampling of reflected ultrasound and accurate range or spatial information.
- PW Doppler spectral displays portray velocity vectors over time. However, the velocity range that can be presented by PW Doppler is limited by the Nyquist limit).

Continuous wave Doppler
Continuous wave (CW) Doppler involves continuous transmission of ultrasound with one transducer element while a second element serves as a receiver.
- Higher sampling rates are achieved, and consequently higher velocities, such as those found in stenotic and regurgitant lesions can be measured.
- CW Doppler does not permit ranging information to be acquired and all velocities along a scan line are included in the spectral trace.

Aliasing and the Nyquist limit

Doppler is restricted in its ability to sample high velocities by the *Nyquist limit* which depends on the sampling rate (the lower the frequency, the higher the evaluable velocity) and object depth (the deeper the object, the lower the sampling rate). When the frequency shift of moving objects (i.e. velocity) exceeds the Nyquist limit, *aliasing* occurs which precludes velocity assessment.

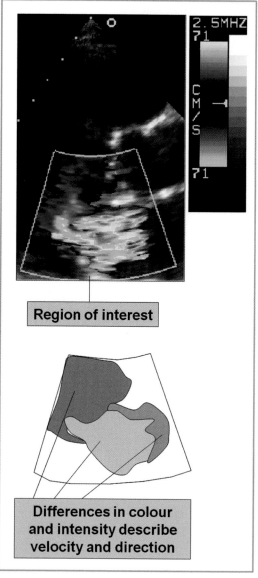

Region of interest

**Differences in colour
and intensity describe
velocity and direction**

Fig. 1.10 Colour flow mapping. In this example colour flow Doppler has been placed across the mitral valve in a parasternal long-axis view to assess mitral regurgitation.

Colour flow Doppler imaging (Fig. 1.8)
Colour flow Doppler imaging employs multigate PW Doppler to portray
blood flow overlying the 2D image. Information is used to detect regurgitant or stenotic lesions or shunts and qualitative assessment of velocities
is possible using colour maps.
- Pixels are assigned a colour based on the scale selected by the user.
  Pixel colour reflects the direction and average velocity in the pixel
  region of interest.
- By convention, the BART colour map system is used (**B**lue represents
  flow **A**way from the transducer and **R**ed represents flow **T**owards the
  transducer). The lighter the colour the higher is the velocity.
- Abnormal velocity distributions characteristic of turbulence can be
  mapped by including a green hue ('variance mapping').
- Aliasing is depicted as a mix of colours or a 'mosaic' pattern.

Tissue Doppler imaging
Tissue Doppler imaging (TDI) is used to assess low-velocity displacement
of structures. A high-pass filter excludes higher-frequency shifts caused by
red cell flow, leaving only low-velocity shifts attributable to wall motion.
- Mitral or tricuspid annular motion can be tracked and correlates with
  systolic and relaxation performance of the associated ventricles.
- Regional wall motion can be assessed for displacement which may be
  affected by overall cardiac motion or local tethering.

Measurements with Doppler

Doppler spectral traces can provide important information regarding flow quantitation (e.g. for assessing valve dysfunction) or timing (e.g. in dyssynchrony studies). The major use of Doppler is for assessing valve function with colour flow mapping used to demonstrate regurgitation, and CW and PW Doppler used to quantify both stenosis and regurgitation. Two key measures obtained with Doppler are pressure gradients across valves and valve area.

Pressure gradients across valves

The velocity of blood cells travelling across a narrow orifice is directly proportional to the pressure gradient at that point in time. This relationship is approximated by the simplified Bernoulli formula:

$$\text{gradient (mmHg)} = 4V^2$$

where V is the peak Doppler velocity (m/s).

In situations where there are high flow velocities (e.g. aortic stenosis with high left ventricular outflow tract (LVOT) velocities) the flow before the stenosis must be accounted for:

$$\text{gradient (mmHg)} = 4(V_2^2 - V_1^2)$$

where V_2 is the velocity across the lesion and V_1 is the pre-lesional velocity).

Both peak and mean gradients can be determined, the latter by integrating the velocity spectra over a cardiac cycle.

Valve area (continuity equation).

This is based on the principle that flow in the pre-valve area (e.g. LVOT) equals the flow across the valve. It is generally used for aortic stenosis quantitation. although it is also applicable to other stenotic orifices.

LVOT flow = LVOT area × LVOT time–velocity integral (TVI)
by PW Doppler

LVOT area = (maximum LVOT diameter in PLA view)^2
aortic valve flow = aortic valve area × aortic valve TVI
by CW Doppler

As aortic valve flow = LVOT flow,

aortic valve area = (LVOT TVI/aortic valve TVI) × LVOT area.

Strain rate imaging and speckle tracking

Strain rate imaging can measure regional thickening and thinning independent of the external influences described above which influence tissue Doppler measurements. With strain rate imaging, two sampling sites are simultaneously acquired and inter-sample displacement (strain) over time (strain rate) can be determined (Fig. 1.11). Speckle tracking uses this principle based on tracking individual speckles within a 2D image (Fig. 1.12).

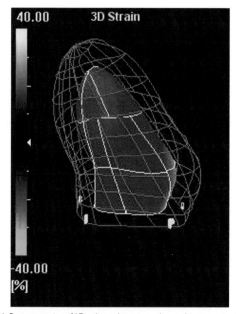

Fig. 1.11 Post-processing of 3D volume datasets can be used to reconstruct a left ventricle and assess function using different parameters including ejection fraction and strain.

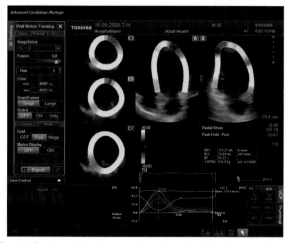

Fig. 1.12 Speckle tracking makes use of inherent speckle within the myocardium. Analysis packages can track these speckles over time to derive indices of strain in two or three dimensions.

Acquisition of transthoracic echocardiography

Images are usually acquired with the patient lying on their left side and stored onto digital media for later review. The ultrasound probe is placed on the chest wall in two standard positions (or windows), the parasternal and apical windows (Fig. 1.13). Further windows can be used as required. A series of 2D images at specific planes through the heart are acquired in each window. These image planes tend to be similar across image modalities. This simplifies recognition and interpretation of structure and pathology. In all views colour flow mapping is also used to assess valves, and then CW and PW Doppler, and occasionally M mode, are used to provide quantitative assessment. 3D, contrast, and tissue Doppler imaging may be needed in some views.

Standard sequence of views

Parasternal window

This window is usually just to the left of the sternum around the third or fourth intercostal space. The first view obtained in echocardiography is usually the long-axis view of the left ventricle and aorta. Rotating the probe by 90° provides a short-axis view (at the level of the aortic valve and then, by rocking the probe, the mitral valve and mid-ventricle). Additional views include the right ventricular inflow/outflow views.

Apical window

As the name suggests this is at the cardiac apex at the bottom left lateral point of the chest. Once the apex is identifed, the different views are obtained by rotating the probe. The key views are the 4-chamber (LV/RV/LA/RA), 5-chamber (as for 4- plus LVOT), 2-chamber (LV/LA), and 3-chamber (as for 2- plus LVOT) views.

Subcostal window

This lies below the xiphisternum in the epigastrium. The patient lies on their back with stomach relaxed and the probe is pointed back up into the chest to look at the cardiac chambers, or directly into the abdomen to look at the inferior vena cava (IVC) and aorta.

Additional windows for views

Suprasternal window

This is the suprasternal notch. The patient lies on their back and raises the chin. This is used to look at the aortic arch.

Right parasternal window

This is used to look at flow in the ascending aorta. The patient lies on their right side and the window is on the right of the sternum, usually slightly higher than the equivalent left parasternal window.

Supraclavicular window

This is rarely needed but can be used to look at vascular structures and the aorta. It lies above the clavicles.

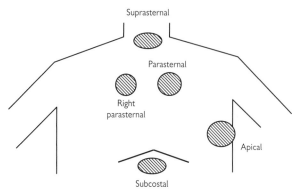

Fig. 1.13 Transthoracic imaging is based on the use of standard acoustic windows on the chest wall to collect all the necessary images.

Transoesophageal echocardiography

Background

Transoesophageal echocardiography (TOE) has emerged over the last 30 years. The first M-mode transoesophageal images were published in the 1970s by Dr Frazin, a cardiologist in Chicago, who attached a traditional probe to the end of an endoscope. By the early 1980s 2D imaging with smaller probe technology was realistic, but the introduction of bi-plane and then multiplane probes provided a leap in functionality. Transoesophageal echocardiography uses the same technology as transthoracic imaging. However, transoesophageal imaging has the major advantage that there is little tissue between the probe and the heart to degrade the image and allows higher ultrasound frequencies to be used (typically 5–7.5MHz) to enhance spatial resolution.

Pathology and TOE

Many of the clinical applications have been driven by interest in intra-operative monitoring and this remains a key application of the technique. However, real-time imaging with unparalleled spatial and temporal resolution makes the technique ideal for detailed assessment of fast-moving and/or small objects such as those found in valve disease. Generally accepted evidence-based uses of transoesophageal echocardiography include:

- haemodynamic monitoring in anaesthetized patients
- evaluation of valve pathology
- intracardiac shunts
- endocarditis
- evaluation of prosthetic valve dysfunction
- congenital heart disease
- aortic dissection and aortic pathology
- cardiac masses (where transthoracic imaging is inadequate)
- imaging during procedures such as percutaneous procedures (ASD/PFO closure, mitral balloon valvotomy, electrophysiology, and pacing), transeptal puncture, lead placement., cardiothoracic surgery.
- poor transthoracic windows or inadequate image quality.

Basics of TOE

The equipment comprises an endoscope fitted with an ultrasound probe on the head. The probe requires cleaning between procedures and/or use of a sheath. The team delivering TOE usually consists of the operator and assistant plus a nurse. The patient is usually sedated and then the probe is intubated down the oeospahagus. The scanhead at the tip of the probe can be moved around 180° to provide multiplane images. By moving the probe up and down, rotating, and angulating inside the oesophagus (and down into the stomach) a range of further image planes can be obtained (Fig. 1.14). A combination of probe movements is required to gather all the images. For many of the views, changes in sector angle are the primary control, with physical movements used to optimize the image.

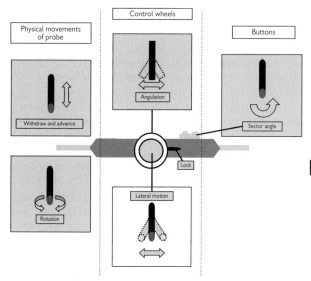

Fig. 1.14 Images in transoesophageal echocardiography are obtained by manipulation of the probe within the oesophagus (left), mechanical movement of the tip of the probe (middle), and rotation of the imaging plane in the tip of the probe (right).

Acquisition
Acquisition of transoesophageal images requires the patient to be in an appropriate position and condition to tolerate insertion of the probe into the oesophagous. It can be performed under sedation with the patient in a lateral decubitus position. If the patient is under general anaesthetic in an intensive care setting or during an operation, the probe is usually inserted with the subject on their back.

Once the probe is positioned images are acquired in a standardized way with a set sequence of views. One approach is to use the screenwiper principle (Fig. 1.15). This is based on altering the angle of the scanner within the probe head to scan through a set of image planes (Box 1.2).

- Starting from 0° the sector is moved across in steps to ~135° and then back again in a series of steps.
- At each step the view needs only minor modifications of probe position to optimize the image. This reduces major probe movements and minimizes patient discomfort.

Each view is examined in:
- 2D imaging
- then colour flow Doppler recordings
- and, if needed, spectral Doppler recordings (pulsed wave and/or continuous wave).

After the screen wiper is complete additional views can be used, as required, to look at pulmonary veins, transgastric views, the aorta, or any abnormal findings.

Basic screenwiper study

1 Four-chamber view
2 Five-chamber view
3 Short-axis aortic view (± right ventricle inflow/outflow)
4 Long-axis aortic view
5 Inter-atrial septal view
6 Left atrial appendage view

Then further views.
7 Left pulmonary venous view
8 Right pulmonary venous view
9 Pulmonary artery view
10 Transgastric views (not necessary in all patients)
11 Descending aorta view
12 Aortic arch view

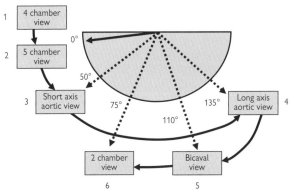

Fig. 1.15 Transoesophageal imaging planes are best obtained by following a standardized sequence of views. The screenwiper principle is a simple approach which ensures systematic collection of the important information.

Three-dimensional echocardiography

Background

If, as well as scanning the ultrasound beam across a linear section of the heart, the entire image plane is scanned up and down, with the echo data fed into a 3D memory array, it is possible to generate a complete data set of the heart's structures rapidly enough to form real-time images. Achievement of this has required overcoming several daunting technological challenges but is now in routine clinical practice. Data display on 2D video screens is achieved by computer-generated texturing and shadowing to emphasize closer structures and create the impression of a 3D solid, which can be rotated and tilted by a trackball and from which individual 2D sections can be extracted. The clinical possibilities for real-time 3D imaging are enormous, particularly in congenital heart disease, and are only just beginning to be explored.

Pathology and 3D echocardiography

3D echocardiography provides opportunities for:
- more precise assessment of ventricular volumes
- multiple image planes for later analysis, including strain analysis, obtained in a single image acquisition
- in transoesophageal imaging, more detailed demonstration the anatomy and pathology of valves, particularly the mitral valve
- in transoesophageal imaging, real-time monitoring in three dimensions of procedures such as occlude device placement and percutaneous valve procedures (Figs 1.16 and 1.17).

Basics of 3D echocardiography

Acquisition requires a 3D probe and an appropriate machine to process the images. The footprint of 3D probes is rapidly reducing in size and most TOE probes now have 3D capabilities. Creating the image follows the same principles as acquiring a 2D image. The region of interest is identified using 2D imaging and then a 3D volume dataset is acquired over one to seven beats. The number of beats determines the image resolution. Real-time imaging is also possible, although the imaging window is usually smaller.

Intracardiac ultrasound

Intracardiac ultrasound probes that can be passed through a sheath placed at a venous access site are now available. These provide a single plane. The tip of the probe can be manipulated and angulated to look at different anatomical areas. Intracardiac ultrasound can be used for percutaneous procedures that would usually require TOE. The use of intra-cardiac ultrasound may allow the procedure to be performed under local rather than general anaesthetic.

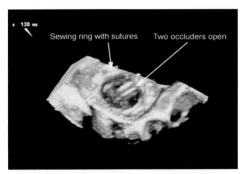

Fig. 1.16 3D echocardiography provides opportunities for real-time 3D visualization of different cardiac structures. This is a transoesophageal echocardiography of a prosthetic mitral valve.

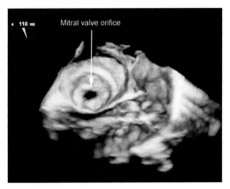

Fig. 1.17 3D transoesophageal echocardiography of the mitral valve viewed from the atrial side with evidence of mitral stenosis.

Cardiovascular magnetic resonance

Background

Nuclear magnetic resonance was first characterized in 1946, and this phenomenon has been utilized through rapid technological developments to provide the high spatial and temporal resolution cardiac images we are familiar with today. The equipment and expertise required to perform cardiovascular magnetic resonance (CMR) has meant that the method has been restricted to a few key centres, but increasingly, as the pool of expertise grows and the equipment becomes more widely available, the technique is being rolled out across different centres. The applications of CMR imaging are also increasing. The introduction of gadolinium-based contrast agents with their ability to image fibrosis within the heart brought CMR into the forefront of ischaemic and congential myocardial assessment. The striking image quality and adaption of CMR for perfusion imaging has further increased the clinical utility of the modality so that it has become an accepted part of routine cardiac care.

Pathology and CMR

The major indication for CMR is assessment of the myocardium in patients with suspected cardiomyopathies. However, it can be used to assess most other areas of cardiac disease as well as to provide information on the vasculature.

- Accurate assessment of left ventricular size, mass, and function, including global and regional left ventricular function. Regional perfusion assessment is also possible.
- Assessment of the myocardium using contrast agents (Fig. 1.18).
- Pericardial disease, in particular thickness.
- Gross cardiopulmonary anatomy.
- Aortic disease.
- Valvular disease, both stenosis and regurgitation, based on flow measures and chamber assessment.

Basics of CMR

Physics

Magnetic resonance depends on the interaction between atomic nuclei and radio waves in the presence of a magnetic field. The major nucleus of interest is the hydrogen atom, which is present throughout the body in water and fat. When the body is placed in a strong magnetic field the hydrogen atoms align themselves in the direction of the field. A radio-frequency wave is then applied to 'knock' some of the hydrogen atoms out of alignment. The hydrogen atoms absorb this radiofrequency energy and then release it as they return to alignment within the field. This energy release is picked up as a signal. The strength and nature of the signal provides information on the hydrogen atoms within different tissues. By altering the number, timing, and features of the radiofrequency pulse an image can be generated.

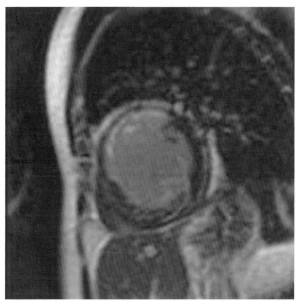

Fig. 1.18 Short-axis CMR image of the left ventricle following injection of gadolinium. This image demonstrates subendocardial enhancement in the anterior wall consistent with a myocardial infarction.

Equipment (Fig. 1.19)

- The key component of a magnetic resonance scanner is the magnet. The higher the magnetic field the more hydrogen atoms will align. A standard clinical scanner has a magnetic flux density of 1.5 Tesla but 3 Tesla systems are increasingly being used. The magnet is constructed by winding wires in rings and cooling them with liquid helium to extremely low temperatures (−269°C) so that they are superconducting. Passing current through the wires then produces the magnetic field. The arrangement of the wires is designed to create a uniform magnetic field within the scanner. Once set up, the magnets are always on even when the scanning console is switched off.
- The other key item is the coils within the scanner which allow a gradient to be generated in the magnetic field. This allows spatial differentiation. The gradient coil lies concentrically within the magnet bore and is controlled by a gradient amplifier.
- The system that emits the radiofrequency pulse comprises a transmit coil, which is usually built into the bore tube, and the receiver coils. These coils are placed on the patient's chest to capture the signal returning from the body. The coils need to be close to the patient and of an appropriate arrangement to pick up the signal. They are usually in a phased array, i.e. they consist of several small coils operated together but receiving signals independently.
- The bed positions the patient within the scanner and ensures that the region of interest is located within the optimal area of the bore.

Gadolinium

Gadolinium contrast has opened the possibility for a range of new sequences with CMR imaging. Gadolinium is an injectable agent which, once fixed to an appropriate carrier, alters the T_1 signal characteristic of any fluid or tissue within which it is present. Therefore it can be used to highlight specific areas. Early imaging allows imaging of movement of the agent through the circulation, and because it can pass out into tissue can also be imaged in areas of scar. It is excreted by the kidneys, and there have been recent concerns about increased incidence of systemic fibrosis following gadolinium injection. This is a fatal irreversible condition and appears to occur in those with severe renal disease in whom, presumably, the gadolinium is not cleared effectively. Gadolinium contrast is contraindicated in severe renal dysfunction.

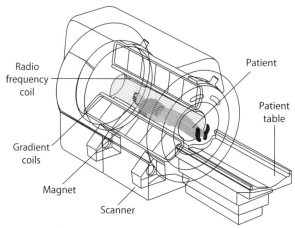

Radio
frequency
coil

Patient

Patient
table

Gradient
coils

Magnet

Scanner

Fig. 1.19 Line drawing of CMR scanner with key components labelled. Reproduced with permission from Myerson SG, Francis J, Neubauer S (2010) *Cardiovascular Magnetic Resonance,* Oxford University Press.

Acquisition

The mangement team for a CMR scan usually comprises radiographers and physicians with expertise in image interpretation and analysis. This team is supported by MR physicists. Once the patient has prepared for the scan and all metallic objects (jewellery etc.) have been removed, they lie on the table and are postioned within the scanner. They have ECG monitoring to allow ECG triggering and wear headphones to block out the noise of the scanner and to communicate with the scanners.

Two broad groups of images are possible:
- static imaging acquired at a fixed point in the cardiac cycle which uses variation in the tissue signal to diagnose cardiac disease
- cine images which provide information on the motion of the heart during the cardiac cycle.

A cardiac scan is then performed. Each image plane is set up by the opera-tor and then the scan is run. Acquisition of each plane usually takes 1–15s depending on the number of cardiac cycles included in the sequence. Acquisition of a standard cardiac scan comprises the following.
- Localizers identify where the subject is within the scanner (usually in several different planes).
- Anatomy—HASTE images, usually in a transverse plane, provide information on cardiac and extracardiac structures.
- Pilots provide static images to orientate the different planes of the heart.
- Cine images generate the standard imaging planes of the heart to assess structure and function (Figs. 1.20 and 1.21).
- Flow imaging provides information on flow across valves or within blood vessels if required.
- Contrast imaging (if required)—this requires injection of gadolinium.
  - Early imaging allows assessment of gadolinium as it passes through the blood vessels and cardiac chambers. Depending on the timing and size of bolus this can be used to perform venography or angiography (e.g. pulmonary vein anatomy), assess myocardial perfusion, or look for thrombus in the left ventricle
  - Late imaging allows assessment of gadolinium that has been retained within tissue and is based on imaging ~5min after the injection. By this time there should be a significant reduction in gadolinium within the blood pool so that any retained contrast should be easy to see. This is used to look for areas of fibrosis such as scarring after myocardial infarction or in hypertrophic cardiomyopathy.
- Further static sequences are possible for looking at tissue characteristics (i.e. turbo spin echo imaging or T_1 or T_2 mapping).
- Perfusion and stress imaging can also be performed.

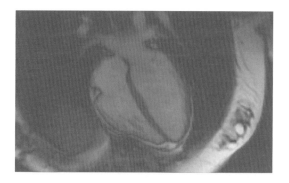

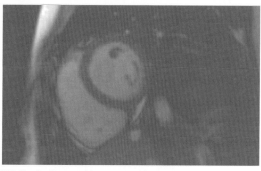

Fig. 1.20 Standard horizontal long-axis views (top) and short-axis views (bottom) of the heart at end-diastole obtained as CMR cine images.

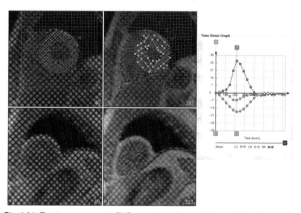

Fig. 1.21 Tagging sequences in CMR generate orthogonal planes within the myocardium at end-diastole. These then deform during systole and the deformation can be tracked with automated analysis software to generate information on systolic strain.

Cardiac computed tomography

Background

Computed tomography (CT) was invented in 1972 by Sir Godfrey Hounsfield and Allan Cormack, and the first clinical CT scanners were installed in 1974. Initial scanners were dedicated to imaging the brain and had a small gantry aperture designed to accommodate only the patient's head. Total body CT scanners with larger gantry apertures were in clinical use by the early 1980s. Today over 40,000 scanners are installed worldwide. Hounsfield and Cormack shared the Nobel Prize for Physiology and Medicine in 1979.

The acquisition of images can be challenging due to small calibre coronary vessels, cardiac contraction and respiratory motion. High temporal resolution (the time needed to acquire a single image without blurring) and small spatial resolution (the ability to discriminate between adjacent structures) is required to overcome these problems. Electron beam CT (EBCT), designed primarily for improved cardiac imaging, was introduced in 1982 but there was poor clinical uptake because of its poor spatial resolution and it is mainly used for coronary calcium scoring. Multi-detector CT scanners and faster gantry rotation has led to improvement in spatial resolution. ECG triggering/gating also improved image quality and reproducibility so that now a complete cardiac CT acquisition is possible in 5–10s.

Pathology and cardiac CT

The major indication for cardiac CT is for coronary artery assessment (Fig. 1.22). However, the quality and quantity of the 'raw' dataset acquired for a coronary CT also allows assessment of other features of cardiac pathology. There are also extended cardiac CT protocols to allow further assessment of cardiac pathology. For a CT coronary angiogram the following can be assessed.

- Gross cardiac anatomy.
- Coronary vessels, including coronary calcification, coronary lumenography and coronary plaque morphology.
- Left ventricle, including global and regional left ventricular function, mass and volume. Identification of areas of fixed hypoperfusion within the left ventricle.
- Assessment of left-sided valvular stenosis assessment in retrospective gated studies.
- Pericardial disease, in particular thickness and calcification.

The extended protocols also allow further assessment of:
- gross cardiopulmonary anatomy;
- more detailed assessment of ventricular size and function including assessment of the right ventricle and detailed studies of left ventricular perfusion;
- further assessment of left- and right-sided valvular stenosis.

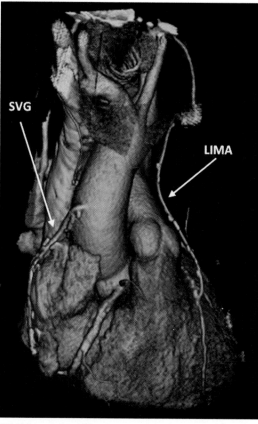

Fig. 1.22 Volume rendered CT coronary angiogram demonstrating left internal mammary artery (LIMA) graft to left anterior descending artery and saphenous vein graft (SVG) to right coronary artery.

Basics of cardiac CT

Equipment

A CT scanner consists of an X-ray tube mounted in a gantry opposite a fixed bank of detectors (64–320). Detectors are usually ~0.5–0.6mm wide (i.e. 320 detectors cover ~16cm). The X-ray tube and detector bank rotate around the patient who is moved through the X-ray beam on the table at a variable speed (pitch). The rotating X-ray tube allows calculation of attenuation at every point within an axial section. This generates a cross-sectional image (of 2D pixels). Moving the patient through the rotating X-ray generates a 3D volumetric dataset (of 3D voxels) from which multiple axial images can be generated (Fig. 1.23).

Several different types of CT scanner are installed in hospitals. The main types are as follows.

Electron beam CT (EBCT)

- X-ray tube mounted in a gantry opposite a fixed detector.
- Excellent temporal resolution (100ms).
- Poor spatial resolution (1mm)^3 precludes CT coronary angiography.
- Rarely used clinically.
- Useful for coronary calcium scoring.

Multi-detector CT (MDCT)

- X-ray tube mounted in a gantry opposite a fixed bank of detectors (64–320).
- Detectors are usually ~0.5–0.6mm wide.
- Choice between wide coverage (i.e. 320 detectors cover ~16cm) or fast acquisition (gemstone detector technology).
- The X-ray tube and detector bank rotate around the patient.
- Temporal resolution = half gantry rotation time (usually 167–250 ms).
- Spatial resolution $(0.3)^3$ mm – $(0.6)^3$ mm.

Dual source CT (DSCT)

- Two X-ray tubes mounted at 90° opposite two fixed banks of detectors (32–128).
- Half the temporal resolution of MDCT as each detector requires a 90° rotation to capture the complete dataset (75–83ms).
- The two detector banks often have different numbers of detectors and different coverage.
- Allows dual energy to be applied but from different spatial orientations.
- Spatial resolution is the same as with MDCT.

Dual energy CT

- DSCT: allows dual energy to be applied but from different spatial orientations.
- Gemstone detector MDCT: changes X-ray energy every 0.4 ms onto fast scintillating detector.
- Both have the potential for digital subtraction (i.e. removal of contrast), negating the need for a non-contrast study prior to the contrast study.
- Not yet used in CT coronary angiography as the spatial resolution is not adequate (p. 44).

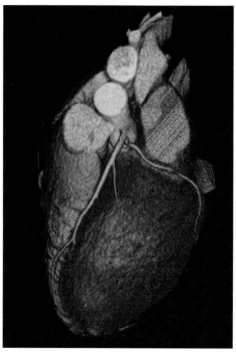

Fig. 1.23 Images of cardiac surface and epicardial coronary vessels obtained from volume-rendered cardiac CT data.

Attenuation: the basis of cardiac CT

The fan-shaped X-ray beam passes through the patient and is attenuated by the organs and anatomical structures that are encountered along its path. The variation in degree of attenuation forms the basis of the creation of the cardiac CT image (Fig. 1.24). Therefore the factors that attenuate the X-ray beam are important as they determine what cardiac CT can image. The key factors are as follows.

- The atomic density of the tissue (the higher the density, the higher the attenuation). Attenuation is measured in Hounsfield units (HU) as an absolute value, where 0 represents water, −1024 represents air, and +1000 represents bone.
- The difference in density between structures within the patient (Table 1.1). The greater the difference in attenuation between adjacent structures, the more readily they can be distinguished.

Anatomical images are generated by combining information on the degree of attenuation from multiple positions (obtained by rotating the gantry). Where there is no intrinsic difference in attenuation between two structures (i.e. between coronary arteries and myocardium), intravascular iodine-based contrast can be used to increase the density of the lumen of the vessel, changing the attenuation and therefore allowing it to be differentiated from surrounding tissue.

Acquisition

The cardiac CT team usually involves a radiographer and a physician experienced in interpretation of cardiac CT. The acquisition protocol usually consists of four separate components.

- Scout scan—used to determine superior and inferior limits of CT acquisition.
- Coronary calcium score—unenhanced CT scan.
- Test bolus—used to determine peak concentration of contrast in the area of interest (aortic root for CT coronary angiogram, pulmonary artery for CT pulmonary angiogram).
- CT coronary angiogram—timing is based on the test bolus. Usually 3–4s is added to allow maximum coronary attenuation.

Table 1.1 Common cardiac structures and their attenuation values in Hounsfield units (HU)

Structure	Attenuation (HU)
Stents	700–1000
Coronary calcium	200–1200
Aortic root	300–500
Coronary lumen	200–400
Coronary vein	150–200
Myocardium	100–200
Fat	0–200

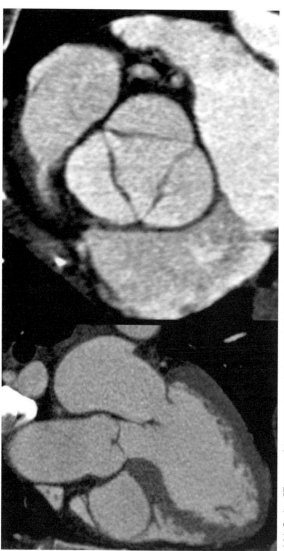

Fig. 1.24 Cardiac CT images of the aortic valve in the long axis (left) and the short axis (right).

CT coronary angiography

MDCT coronary angiography (CTA) (Figs. 1.25–1.27) has been compared with invasive coronary angiography at each stage of development. The real strength of CTA is its negative predictive value, i.e. its ability to exclude coronary artery disease. 64-detector data suggest a sensitivity of 99% and specificity of 95% with a negative predictive value of 99%. The positive predictive value of CTA in technically adequate studies varies between 50% and 90% in major multicentre studies.

CTA should be considered in those patients:
• with low to intermediate pre-test probability of significant coronary artery disease;
• who do not wish to have an invasive coronary angiogram;
• in whom an invasive coronary angiogram is likely to be problematic (i.e. severe peripheral vascular disease);
• in whom there is a high likelihood of aberrant coronary vessels (i.e. in adult congenital heart disease);
• in those where the risk of invasive coronary angiogrpahy is particularly high (i.e. severe aortic stenosis);
• in whom an alternative to myocardial perfusion scintigraphy is sought.

MDCT should not be carried out on patients with a high risk of coronary artery disease since invasive angiography can and should lead seamlessly into immediate intervention in this group.

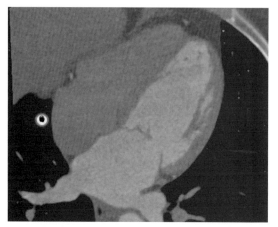

Fig. 1.25 Axial CT coronary angiogram dataset demonstrating left anterior descending (LAD), right coronary (RCA), and left circumflex obtuse marginal (OM) arteries and clear mitral valve opening.

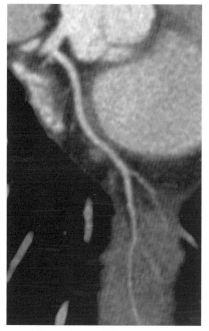

Fig. 1.26 Curved multiplanar reformatted CT coronary angiogram dataset demonstrating left main stem and left circumflex artery.

Coronary calcium scoring

The prevalence and extent of coronary calcium varies widely and increases with age in both men and women. Even small quantities of coronary calcium have a significant impact on prognosis and mortality. The presence of coronary calcium almost always represents atherosclerosis, and screening is particularly beneficial in reclassifying individuals at intermediate clinical risk. Calcium burden represents only one-fifth of total coronary plaque burden and there is no one-to-one correlation between calcified lesion in the coronary artery and underlying significant stenosis. Furthermore, the locationS of coronary calcium and any stenosis present are often different. Coronary calcium can be scored using different scanners.

EBCT assessment utilizes the Agatston calcium score, which is the sum of all calcium clusters within all coronary arteries, adjusted for peak density, giving an overall figure. Calcification is identified on the unenhanced scan using a 130HU threshold. All calcific lesions with an area >1mm^2 are scored.

MDCT, like EBCT, accurately identifies coronary calcium and allows direct quantification of the overall burden of disease. MDCT utilizes a modified version of this score; the Agatston score equivalent (ASE), but can additionally provide volumetric and mass quantification. Patients are usually classified as having minimal (ASE 1–10), mild (ASE 11–100), moderate (ASE 101–400), or severe (ASE >400) coronary calcification.

A coronary calcium scan requires <1mSv of radiation and usually forms part of MDCT coronary angiographic protocols prior to contrast injection. High levels of coronary calcium may prevent full assessment via MDCT coronary angiography because of overprojection of high-density plaque into the lumen. Therefore a known high calcium score is a relative contraindication to MDCT coronary angiography.

Population screening

Coronary calcium scoring is unproven as a population screening tool. By comparing the total ASE with that of others of the same age and gender through the use of a large database of asymptomatic patients a calcium percentile is derived and gives an index of atherosclerosis. Ethnic variation may exist but is not currently incorporated into these nomograms and so caution should be applied in the non-Caucasian population.

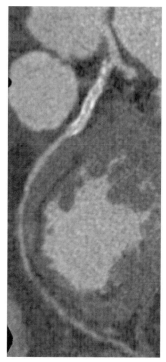

Fig. 1.27 Curved multiplanar reformatted CT coronary angiogram dataset demonstrating a coronary stent in the LAD.

Myocardial perfusion scintigraphy

Background
Nuclear cardiology encompasses any technique that relies on the decay of a radioactive particle which is then detected and processed into a recognizable image. Nuclear techniques can be used to label the blood pool (to measure ventricular function) and to label myocardial cells or blood flow (to measure viability or ischaemia). The nomenclature can be confusing, especially as the most available technique within nuclear cardiology is known by many names, including the name of the isotope:

Positron emission tomography (PET) relies on a different set-up and type of detection system. Cardiac PET is limited to a few centres and is predominantly used in a research setting, although clinical applications are increasing predominantly on the back of PET/CT expansion in oncology.

Pathology and myocardial perfusion scintigraphy
There is a vast body of data going back over 30 years looking at all aspects of nuclear perfusion imaging. Large-scale studies with long-term follow-up are common. The major use is to diagnose coronary artery disease. Every tracer and method of stress has been tested. The diagnostic and prognostic value of myocardial perfusion scintigraphy (MPS) has been established (Figs. 1.28–1.30). The published sensitivity is >90% with a similar normalcy rate. Groups that are difficult to assess, such as the elderly, diabetics, women, and those with conduction defects, have all been found to benefit from strategies utilizing MPS.

The prognostic value of a normal scan is excellent, with a major cardiovascular event rate of <1% over at least 5 years. Similarly, an abnormal scan can be risk stratified according to the size and extent of defect present. The greater the size of the defect the worse is the prognosis. Reversible defects constituting >12% of the myocardium are likely to benefit from revascularization over medical therapy. Left ventricular function assessment increases the prognostic value. Therefore indications include the following.
- Diagnose coronary artery disease.
- Heart failure assessment—hibernation and diagnosing coronary artery disease.
- Pre non-cardiac surgery to assess risk.
- Pre revascularization to identify coronary target lesions.
- Post revascularization to determine post-procedural reduction in ischaemia.
- Acute chest pain when there has been a non-diagnostic ECG.
- Post acute coronary syndrome to risk stratify.

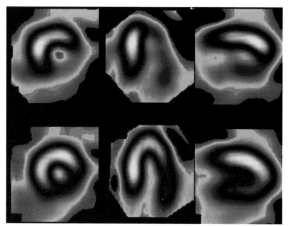

Fig. 1.28 Myocardial perfusion scintigraphy planes after stress (top row) and at rest (bottom row). The images demonstrate evidence of inducible ischaemia in an inferolateral territory.

Names in nuclear cardiology

The techniques employed in nuclear cardiology are:
• planar imaging
• single-photon emission computed tomography (SPECT)
• radionuclide ventriculography (RNV) sometimes erroneously called 'MUGA scan'.

Myocardial perfusion scintigraphy (MPS) is also known as:
• myocardial perfusion imaging (MPI)
• nuclear perfusion scan
• 'thallium' scan—named after the first widespread radio-isotope
• 'Mibi' scan—contracted from technetium-99m sestamibi (Cardiolite™)
• 'Myoview' scan—from technetium-99m tetrofosmin (Myoview™).

Basics of myocardial perfusion scintigraphy

Radioactive decay

Nuclear cardiology relies on the decay of radioactive particles. There are three types of decay: alpha (α), beta (β), and gamma (γ). Nuclear medicine relies predominantly on gamma.

- Decay is measured in becquerels (Bq) with 1Bq equivalent to one decay per second. Technetium-99m has a half-life of 6h and therefore after one day (24h or 4 half-lives) the activity of the sample will be ~6% of the original sample.
- However, the effective half-life of a radioactive isotope is also related to the biological half-life which depends on the metabolism and excretion of the isotope. Therefore the effective half-life may be shorter than the physical half-life if the agent is excreted rapidly.
- Equivalent absorbed radiation dose is measured in sieverts (Sv). It is essentially 'corrected' for the type of radiation emitted and therefore is more useful than the absorbed radiation dose (measured in grays (Gy)). The radiation effective dose is the sum of all the tissue-weighted effective doses and is also expressed in sieverts.

Radiopharmaceuticals

The two main radiopharmaceutical agents use technetium-99m (^{99m}Tc) eluted from a portable on-site generator. It is bound to a commercial product, either sestamibi (Cardiolite™) or tetrofosmin (Myoview™), prior to injection.

^{99m}Tc has a physical half-life of 6h (effective dose equivalent of 8–10mSv per 1000MBq injection). Agents passively diffuse across cell membranes and fix within viable myocardial cells (<2% enters the myocardium). Separate 'stress' and 'rest' injections are required, done as a 1- or 2-day protocol. The agents are excreted by the biliary and renal route and there is also gut uptake of tracer, which can impair image quality.

Thallium-201 (^{201}Tl) is produced in a cyclotron and decays to mercury-201, emitting a combination of γ rays and X-rays (68–80keV). The physical half-life is 73h with an effective dose equivalent of 14mSv per 80MBq injection. No preparation is required apart from producing the correct aliquots. Because it is a K^+ analogue it depends on the Na^+–K^+ channel to enter the cell and 5% of the dose initially enters the myocardium. 'Stress' imaging is performed after 5–15min and then the agent is allowed to redistribute within the blood pool over the next 4h after which the 'rest' acquisition is taken. In critical disease redistribution can be delayed by up to 24h. The agent is excreted by the renal route.

Which agent is best?

There is no correct answer as no tracer is ideal. However, each agent has certain characteristics which lend it to a particular type of study. Overall ^{99m}Tc agents are probably better suited to the standard day-to-day patient undergoing ischaemia testing. ^{201}Tl is slightly more technically challenging to use but is probably superior when it comes to detecting viable/hibernating myocardium (Fig 1.29).

Technetium-99m

- Multiple acquisitions possible, which can reduce artefacts.
- Photon energy ideally suited to gamma cameras.
- ECG gated acquisition allows functional analysis.
- Superior image quality.
- Lower overall dose with shorter half-life.
- Probably more user friendly.
- Recent problems with supply from nuclear reactors.

Thallium-201

- Superior extraction fraction.
- Lung uptake provides incremental prognostic value.
- Viability assessment likely to be superior.

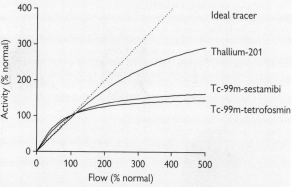

Fig. 1.29 Relationship between absolute myocardial perfusion (flow) and tracer uptake activity) for the three radiopharmaceuticals used in myocardial perfusion scintigraphy (graph not to scale).

Radiation protection

Exposure

Radiation exposes cells to energy deposition and subsequent ionization. Free radicals are commonly produced, resulting in cellular damage. Direct damage to DNA is less common. The effects can be divided into acute and late effects.

Acute effects

The likelihood of acute effects is deterministic, i.e. there is a threshold above which effects occur. The severity of the effect is directly related to the dose received above this threshold. Problems typically arise when dose is >500mSv. For comparison, MPS doses vary from 8 to 20mSv (Table 1.2).

Late effects

Late effects are stochastic, i.e. they do not depend on exceeding a specific threshold. Therefore there is an increased probability of effects with increased doses. However, the severity of the occurrence is not proportional to the dose and therefore there is no safe lower radiation exposure dose. The overriding principle is As Low As Reasonably Achievable (ALARA).

Protection

The principles of radiation minimization and protection are based on minimizing time and maximizing distance and shielding. For staff this means training to avoid exposure by using lead-screened sources. Lead aprons are not necessary for ionizing radiation at this level and are not routinely worn. Dosimeters are worn and analysed on a monthly basis to monitor individual exposure. The requirements for patients are as follows.

- Drink plenty of fluid and pass urine frequently to expel the radio-isotope.
- Avoid prolonged contact with pregnant women or children for 24h after the scan.
- Normal interactions should continue.
- Airport radiation detectors may be activated for up to 3 days.

Clearly pregnant women should not undergo MPS.

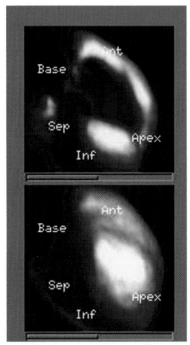

Fig. 1.30 3D volume reconstructions of MPS data after stress (top) and at rest (bottom). An anterolateral inducible defect is evident.

Table 1.2 Risk of cancer induction associated with radiopharmaceutical protocols used in MPS

Radio-pharmaceutical	Protocol	Dose (MBq)	Effective dose equivalent (mSv)	Lifetime risk of fatal cancer
Thallium-201	Stress redistribution	80	14	1 in 1429
	Stress-reinjection	120	21	1 in 952
99mTc-sestamibi	2 day	800	8	1 in 2500
	1 day	1000	10	1 in 2000
99mTc-tetrofosmin	2 day	800	6	1 in 3333
	1 day	1000	8	1 in 2667

Reproduced with permission from Sabharwal N, Loong CY, and Kelion A (2008) *Nuclear Cardiology*, Oxford University Press.

Equipment

Current gamma cameras are based on a sodium iodide (NaI) crystal that scintillates when exposed to a photon of energy. This technology has been unchanged from the 1960s until relatively recently. There are two main types of gamma camera.

The Anger camera

The patient lies or sits on a gantry around which the gamma camera is placed. Photons that escape from the body first encounter a lead collimator which is effectively a lens. Only photons perpendicular to the collimator are allowed through to the NaI crystal.

These photons interact with the crystal and emit a visible light which is detected and amplified by photomultiplier tubes (PMTs) at the back of the camera. The resultant electrical signal is transmitted to a computer workstation.

The position of the camera relative to the body is known and therefore the path of the photon is back-projected to its origin within the myocardium onto a digital matrix.

Simultaneous ECG gated acquisition allows up to 32 time points to be recorded between each R wave and added to the digital matrix. This allows functional assessment.

Solid state detector camera

New solid state crystal detectors, using compounds such as caesium zinc telluride, have been developed which are more accurate, are faster, and have fewer components. These new solid state cameras are a revolutionary step forwards.

- SPECT acquisition is reduced from 15 to 2min.
- Radiation dose can be significantly reduced.
- Motion and attenuation artefacts are reduced.
- Myocardial blood flow quantitation is available (not yet licensed).
- Patient throughput is increased.
- The addition of 64 detector cardiac CTA promises perfusion, function, and anatomical correlation at a relatively low radiation dose.

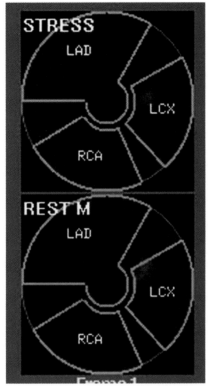

Fig. 1.31 Polar views generated to simplify interpretation of nuclear cardiology data on perfusion.

Acquisition

There are two types of image acquisition: planar and SPECT.

Planar

Planar acquisition involving fixed position gamma camera heads is no longer routinely performed. Prior to the development of rotating SPECT gamma cameras, this technique was employed to image the LV myocardium in fixed planes. Fewer counts are needed using SPECT imaging.

SPECT

This technique relies on a rotating gamma camera which detects photons in a 3D manner. This allows images to be reorientated according to orthogonal axes and allows comparison with other techniques such as echocardiography and CMR (Fig. 1.31).

Increasing the number of rotating gamma camera heads allows more counts to be detected and reduces the acquisition time. Two- or three-headed gamma cameras are now the norm.

Problems during image acquisition

Most problems with image acquisition are related to technical issues rather than patient selection. On the whole there is no absolute contraindication to nuclear perfusion imaging in any patient. Nevertheless problems can occur in the following scenarios.

- Patient movement during scan acquisition:
  - rescan or attenuation correction may be required.
- Not enough radioactivity injected in very obese patients.
- Increased heart rate variability (e.g. poorly controlled atrial fibrillation) can affect ECG gated acquisition:
  - left ventricular ejection fractions (LVEFs) should be interpreted with caution.

Radionuclide ventriculography (RNV)

Background

There are many terms in current use for this technique of assessing ventricular function by radiolabelling the blood pool. Probably, and erroneously, the most commonly used term is MUGA scan.

Pathology and radionuclide ventriculography
- Global LVEF.
  - Especially serial monitoring.
- Regional LV function.
- RVEF.
  - "First pass" or SPECT only.
- Accurate monitoring of cardiotoxic therapy.
  - Anthracyclines or Trastuzumab.
- Exercise RNV can be used in the following situations:
  - Asymptomatic severe aortic regurgitation.
  - Pre non cardiac surgery (risk assessment).
  - Assessment of risk in heart failure.

Basics of radionuclide ventriculography
Technique
- Red blood cells are radiolabelled with ^{99m}Tc-pertechnetate (either *in vitro* or *in vivo*).
- The injected radioactivity is then detected, using a planar approach, either "first pass" or by "equilibrium".
- Counts are gated over 16-32 frames to produce regional and global LVEF.
- A SPECT based algorithm is now available which produces LVEF & RVEF with an "equilibrium" method.

Problems
- Non radiation based alternatives.
- Technical expertise required.
- LVEF also provided by MPS SPECT.

Positron emission tomography (PET)

Background
Cardiac PET is predominantly a research-based tool. However, there has recently been an increase in interest based on the expansion in provision through oncology.

Pathology and PET
- Perfusion imaging:
  - allows absolute flow quantitation (mL/min/g)
- Hibernation and ischaemia assessment:
  - number of viable segments correlates well with the improvement in LVEF post revascularization.

Basics of PET
Technique
- Higher-energy photon pairs (512keV) are emitted by positron-releasing radionuclides
- These photons travel perpendicularly to each other and are registered using coincidence detection
- A cyclotron is usually required (except for rubidium).

Radionuclides
- For flow/perfusion:
  - ^{13}N-ammonia (from an on-site cyclotron)
  - ^{82}Rb (from a commercial generator—lasts 4 weeks).
- For metabolism/viability:
  - ^{18}F-FDG.

Problems
- Very few centres performing cardiac studies.
- Diabetics have extra problems with hibernation assessment using ^{18}F-FDG.
- Currently ^{82}Rb is very expensive compared with SPECT isotopes.
- On-site cyclotron required for ^{13}N-ammonia production.

The future
- Likely to become more popular but unlikely to overtake SPECT.
- Addition of 64 detector cardiac CTA promises perfusion, function, and anatomical correlation at a relatively low radiation dose.

Chapter 2

Imaging planes

Imaging planes *64*
Long axis: four-chamber view *66*
Long axis: five-chamber view *68*
Long axis: two-chamber view (LV) *70*
Long axis: two-chamber view (RV) *72*
Long axis: three-chamber view *74*
Short axis: aortic valve view *76*
Short axis: mitral valve view *78*
Short axis: left ventricular view *80*
Right ventricular inflow view *82*
Right ventricular outflow view *84*
Inferior vena cava views *86*
Aortic views *88*
Pulmonary vein views *90*
Coronary sinus views *90*
Polar view *92*
3D reconstructions *94*

Imaging planes

Body imaging planes

The first sets of planes to become familiar with are those that divide up the body. These are best described by assuming that the body is standing upright and facing towards you. Any particular plane can occur at any point through the body along the axis of the plane, and therefore is also usually referenced according to some anatomical landmark (e.g a vertebral body) or distance from that landmark. The basic planes can be described as follows.

- Transverse—these are horizontal planes, the classic cross-sectional CT view (Fig. 2.1). They can be referenced to a landmark, although in some imaging modalities the images are labelled according to fixed points within the scanner. When displayed they are viewed as if looking from the feet.
- Coronal—up and down, with the body cut from left to right, as if looking straight at the whole body (Fig. 2.1). The classic coronal view is the view of the two hemispheres of the brain or a slice through both kidneys.
- Sagittal—up and down, with the body cut from front to back (Fig. 2.1). The classic sagittal view is the slice down the vertebral column.
- Oblique sagittal—as for sagittal but at a slight angle from the true front to back axis. The classic oblique sagittal view is the slice through the arch and descending aorta.

Cardiac imaging planes

Body image planes allow an overview of anatomy. The standard structures of the heart are not clearly displayed with these imaging planes and therefore there are additional cardiac imaging planes. Fortunately, the same planes are used across modalities, although they often have slightly different names between modalities. They can be grouped into four broad groups.

- Long axis—these lie along the long axis of the structure you are interested in i.e. the plane that gives the longest dimension of the object. For example a long axis of the heart is (an axis parallel to the septum that passes through the apex) These views provide information on cardiac chambers and valve leaflets and include the apical four-chamber view or left ventricular outflow view
- Short axis—these planes lie roughly perpendicular to the long axis at the structure you are interested in and display the heart in cross section. They can lie at any point in the heart to highlight particular structures (e.g. short axis of the left ventricle, aortic valve, or mitral valve).
- Miscellaneous—a range of specialized views that have been developed to allow particular structures to be seen such as the atrial septum or pulmonary veins.
- Polar—these are designed to display the whole left ventricle as a map with the apex at the centre.

Coronary imaging planes are distinct from other imaging modalities and therefore are discussed separately in the section on this imaging modality, page 8. Chest X-ray is essentially a coronal view of the chest.

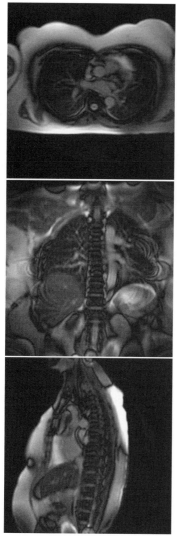

Fig. 2.1 Cardiovascular magnetic resonance pilot images demonstrating transverse (top), coronal (middle), and sagittal (bottom) planes.

Long axis: four-chamber view

This allows assessment of overall left and right ventricular function as well as right and left ventricular inflow.

Names

- Echo—apical four-chamber view
- TOE—0° four chamber view
- CMR—horizontal long axis (HLA)
- CT—not often acquired
- Nuclear—four chamber long-axis view

The view (Fig. 2.2)

The optimal image should extend from the apex (the true apex is identified by the fact that it moves less than the other walls and is thinner). In a true unforeshortened view the left ventricle will be at its longest. Both ventricles, both atria, and both mitral and tricuspid valves should be visible. Septa should be straight down the centre of the image.

Sometimes it is difficult to get both the atria and the ventricles in full view. In this case the image can be optimized based on the area of the heart of interest, usually the ventricles.

What do you see?

Mitral valve

A2 and P2 segments of mitral valve are seen, which allow assessment of movement. Lateral and septal mitral valve annulus is also visible.

Tricuspid valve

Lateral and septal leaflets displayed.

Left and right atrium

Both atria and the inter-atrial septum can be seen. Pulmonary veins as well as vena cavae may also be visible. Can be used to measure atrial size.

Left ventricle

Key view for studying global and regional left ventricular function. Septum, apex, and lateral wall are displayed.

Right ventricle

A key view for looking at the right ventricle size and function. Usually compared with the left ventricle, but quantitative measures are also possible.

Pericardium

Important view for seeing size and location of pericardial fluid.

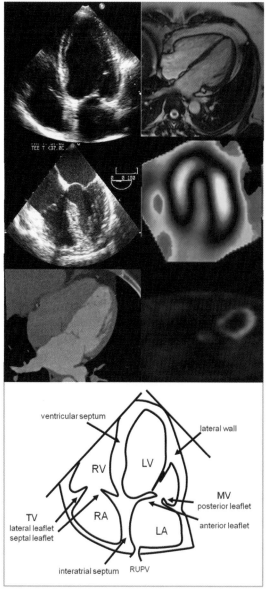

Fig. 2.2 Four-chamber (or horizontal long-axis) views of the heart.

Long axis: five-chamber view

Used to look at the left ventricular outflow and the aortic valve.

Names
- Echo—apical five-chamber view
- TOE—0° five-chamber or 0° deep transgastric view
- CT/nuclear—not often acquired
- CMR—usually acquired as a three chamber LVOT view (p. 74)

The view (Fig. 2.3)
The optimal image looks similar to that obtained with the long-axis four-chamber view, but adjusted to include the aortic valve and ascending aorta.

What do you see?
Aortic valve
Right and non-coronary cusps (although they may not be easy to see).

Left ventricular outflow tract
During echocardiography used with colour flow mapping for aortic regurgitation or flow turbulence due to obstruction. Best view to place pulsed wave Doppler to assess outflow and obstruction.

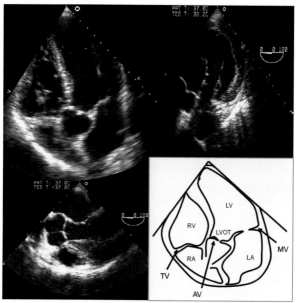

Fig. 2.3 Echocardiographic five chamber view demonstrating transthoracic
(top left), 0° in oesophagus (bottom left), and deep transgastric transoesophageal
(top right) echocardiography.

Long axis: two-chamber view (LV)

An important view for global and regional left ventricular assessment.

Names
- Echo—Apical two chamber view
- TOE—90° two-chamber or transgastric 90° view
- CMR—vertical long-axis (VLA) view
- Nuclear—two-chamber long-axis view
- CT—not often acquired

The view (Fig. 2.4)
The optimal image shows the left ventricle (no right ventricle) from the apex, centred in the image. The mitral valve is cut through the commissure. The left atrium is seen with left atrial appendage visible.

What do you see?
Left ventricle
Inferior wall and anterior wall (closest to left atrial appendage). Good for regional assessment. Used for ventricular volume and function measures.

Mitral valve
The ideal image is a commissural view with P3, A2, and P1 segments visible. It is possible to assess the long axis of the mitral valve annulus.

Left atrial appendage
This is sometimes visible as a curved finger pointing round the side of the mitral valve.

Coronary sinus
The coronary sinus is usually seen in cross section on the opposite side of the mitral valve from the left atrial appendage.

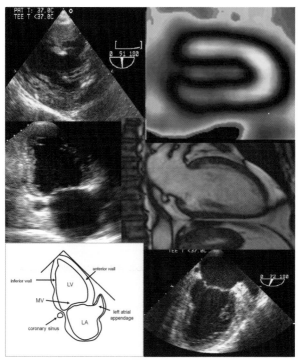

Fig. 2.4 Two-chamber (or vertical long-axis) views of the heart. TOE transgastric (top left) nuclear perfusion (top right) transthoracic (middle left), CMR (middle right), TOE oesophageal (bottom right).

Long axis: two-chamber view (RV)

This view is used to assess right ventricular appearance.

Names
- Echo—apical two-chamber view of right ventricle
- TOE—Transgastric 90° RV two-chamber view
- CMR—Right ventricle vertical long axis (RV VLA)
- Nuclear—not often acquired
- CT—not often acquired

The view (Fig. 2.5)
The optimal image shows the right ventricle (no left ventricle) from the apex, centred in the image. The tricuspid valve is cut through with papillary muscles evident. Inferior and superior vena cavae may be seen.

What do you see?
Right ventricle
This can be used for regional assessment of the inferior and anterior parts of the free wall. Because of the variable anatomy of the right ventricle and the fact it curves around the left ventricle, overall assessment is difficult.

Tricuspid valve
This can be a useful image to look at the subvalvular apparatus, particularly in TOE.

Inferior and superior vena cavae
These may also be seen to assess inflow.

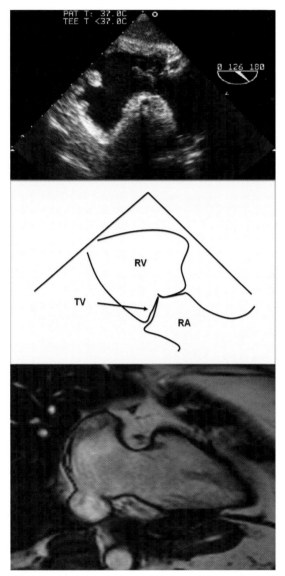

Fig. 2.5 Right ventricular two-chamber (or vertical long-axis) views of the heart using transoeosphageal echocardiography (top) and cardiovascular magnetic resonance (bottom).

Long axis: three-chamber view

This view is mainly used to assess the left ventricular outflow.

Names

- Echo—parasternal long-axis view; apical three-chamber view.
- TOE—135° aortic valve long-axis view
- CMR—left ventricular outflow tract
- CT—not often acquired
- Nuclear—not often acquired

The view (Fig. 2.6)

The optimal image cuts through the middle of mitral and aortic valves to display left ventricular inflow and outflow. The left ventricle is seen extending to the apex. The ascending aorta is seen as a tube with parallel walls.

Sometimes not all structures are seen in a single view and multiple views are collected with a focus on different details.

What do you see?

Left ventricle

The septum (anteroseptal portion), inferolateral wall, and cavity are seen. The wall (in particular the septum) and left ventricular outflow tract can be assessed for size and evidence of obstruction.

Aortic valve

The right coronary cusp is closest to the septum and the non-coronary cusp closest to left atrium. Can be used to assess opening of valve.

Aortic root

The entire aortic root, including sinuses, sinotubular junction, and ascending aorta, should be visible.

Ascending aorta

The proximal portion of the ascending aorta is visible.

Descending aorta

This is seen in cross section as a circle behind the mitral valve.

Mitral valve

The A2 and P2 segments are usually seen. Cine loops allow assessment of movement (prolapse, stenosis, etc.).

Left atrium

The left atrial diameter can be measured.

Right ventricle

The right ventricle is not always well seen but some portion of it will be visible close to the septum and aortic valve.

Pericardium

This is evident anteriorly in front of the right heart and posteriorly behind heart. Effusions should be evident if present.

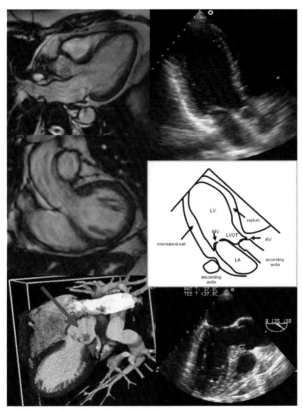

Fig. 2.6 Left ventricular outflow tract views. Left: CMR standard view similar to the three-chamber echocardiographic view (top), CMR coronal LVOT view (taken at 90° to the other CMR view (middle), and a cardiac CT reconstructed view to demonstrate the left ventricular outflow (bottom). Right: transthoracic three-chamber echocardiography view (top) and transoesophageal 135° long-axis view of the aortic valve and the LVOT (bottom).

Short axis: aortic valve view

The short axis view of the aortic valve is the classic Y-shaped cross sectional view.

Names
- Echo—parasternal short-axis aortic valve
- TOE—50° oesophageal short-axis aortic valve
- CMR—short-axis aortic valve
- CT—not often acquired
- Nuclear—not often acquired

The view (Fig. 2.7)
The optimal image should have a round aortic valve with three cusps evident. The tricuspid valve and pulmonary valve should be visible.

What do you see?
Aortic valve
Lies in the centre with the classic Y-shape of left, right, and non-coronary cusps. Left main stem sometimes seen by left cusp.

Right ventricle
The basal right ventricle lies wrapped around the aortic valve. The ventricle can be measured.

Tricuspid valve
Seen beside the aortic valve.

Pulmonary valve
Lies on the other side of the aortic valve from the tricuspid valve.

Left atrium
Lies behind the aortic valve.

Inter-atrial septum
The septum lies between the left and right atria and extends up to the aortic root.

Pericardium
Seen best around the right heart.

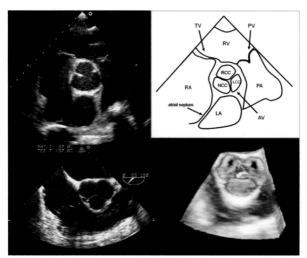

Fig. 2.7 Short-axis aortic valve level: transthoracic parasternal echocardiography (top left) and transoesophageal 50° oesophageal view (bottom left). Note that these views are mirror images. The bottom right image is a 3D transoesophageal view with colour flow to demonstrate central aortic regurgitation.

Short axis: mitral valve view

The short axis view of the mitral valve is the classic 'fish mouth' cross-sectional view of the mitral valve

Names
- Echo—parasternal short-axis mitral valve level
- TOE—transgastric 0° short-axis mitral valve level
- CMR—short-axis mitral valve, short-axis basal slice
- CT—not often acquired
- Nuclear—not often acquired

The view (Fig. 2.8)
The optimal image should have the mitral valve with both leaflets evident.

What do you see?

Mitral valve
This lies in the centre with the classic 'fish mouth' shape.

Right ventricle and tricuspid valve
The basal right ventricle or tricuspid valve may be seen adjacent to the mitral valve.

Left ventricular outflow
The left ventricular outflow may sometimes come in and out of view because of the mobility of this basal slice.

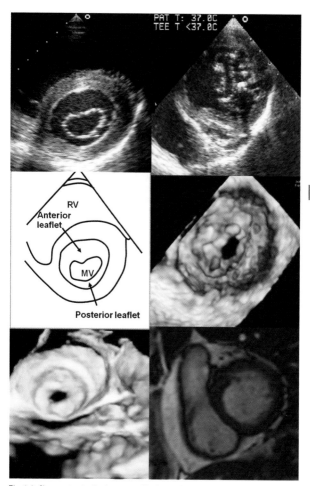

Fig. 2.8 Short-axis mitral valve views. Clockwise from top left: transthoracic echocardiography parasternal short-axis view; transoesophageal echocardiography transgastric 90° short-axis view; 3D transoesophageal echocardiography viewed from the ventricular side of the valve; cardiac magnetic resonance basal slice and 3D transoesophageal echocardiography viewed from the atrial side of the valve.

Short axis: left ventricular view

The short-axis views can be thought of as cross-sectional views through the left ventricle to assess function and size.

Names
- Echo—parasternal short axis,
- TOE—transgastric 0° short-axis left ventricle level
- CMR—short-axis left ventricle or short-axis stack
- CT—not often acquired
- Nuclear—short-axis left ventricle

The view (Fig. 2.9)
The optimal image should have a round left ventricle with the right heart as a crescent wrapped around the right ventricle. The short-axis view can be obtained at different levels and therefore will contain different proportions of the papillary muscles depending on the level.

What do you see?
Left ventricle
Any segment of the left ventricle depending on the choice of level. Papillary muscles will also be seen.

Right ventricle
Seen as a crescent around the side of the left ventricle.

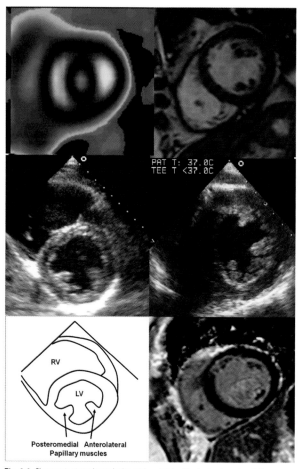

Fig. 2.9 Short-axis view through the mid-ventricle. Clockwise from top left: images generated with nuclear perfusion, cardiovascular magnetic resonance, trans-oesophageal echocardiography, cardiovascular magnetic resonance with gadolinium contrast, and transthoracic echocardiography.

Right ventricular inflow view

A useful view for looking at the tricuspid valve and right ventricular inflow.

Names
- Echo—parasternal right ventricular inflow view
- TOE—bicaval view
- CMR—right ventricular inflow view, right ventricular VLA
- CT—not often acquired
- Nuclear—not often acquired

The view (Fig. 2.10)
The optimal image demonstrates the tricuspid valve with the right atrium behind and sometimes vena caval inflow.

What do you see?
Tricuspid valve
Main feature: two leaflets seen in centre of screen.

Right atrium
May see right atrial appendage, Eustachian valve, and inflow from vena cavae.

Right ventricle
Portion of right ventricle close to tricuspid valve can be seen.

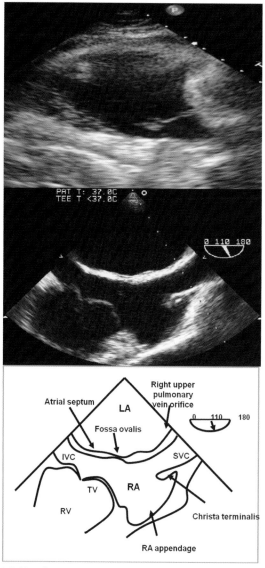

Fig. 2.10 Views for studying right ventricular inflow: parasteranl transthoracic view optimized to view the inflow (top), and a transoesophageal 110° bicaval view which includes the septum, superior vena cava, and in this instance the tricuspid valve (bottom).

Right ventricular outflow view

A useful view for looking at the pulmonary valve and artery.

Names
- Echo—parasternal right ventricular outflow view
- TOE—40° pulmonary artery view
- CMR—right ventricular outflow view, pulmonary artery view
- CT—not often acquired
- Nuclear—not often acquired

The view (Fig. 2.11)
The optimal image demonstrates the pulmonary valve with the pulmonary arterial trunk as far as bifurcation.

What do you see?
Pulmonary valve
Main feature: two leaflets seen.

Pulmonary artery
This can often be seen as far as bifurcation and can be used to measure size and look for abnormal jets (patent ductus) or thrombus (pulmonary embolus).

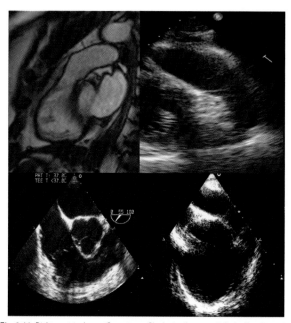

Fig. 2.11 Right ventricular outflow views. Clockwise from top left the first image is a right ventricular outflow view on cardiovascular magnetic resonance in which the plane has been set as an oblique sagittal plane through the pulmonary artery and into the right ventricle. The next image is a parasternal transthoracic echocardiographic view in which the probe has been tilted upwards from a long-axis view to focus on the right ventricular outflow. At 40° in the oesophagus, transoesophageal echocardiography can identify the pulmonary artery, and at 70° when at the level of the aortic valve it shows details of the pulmonary valve.

Inferior vena cava views

These views can be useful to help assess right atrial pressure

Names

- Echo—subcostal inferior vena caval view
- TOE—not often acquired
- CMR—right ventricular inflow view, caval view
- CT—not often acquired
- Nuclear—not often acquired

The view (Fig. 2.12)

The optimal image is a portion of the inferior vena cava inserting into the right atrium. Sometimes the superior vena cava can be included in the same view. Hepatic veins may be seen emptying into the inferior vena cava.

What do you see?

Inferior vena cava

Used to measure diameter and whether it reduces in size with inspiration (normally it should do).

Liver and hepatic veins

These can be seen draining into the inferior vena cava.

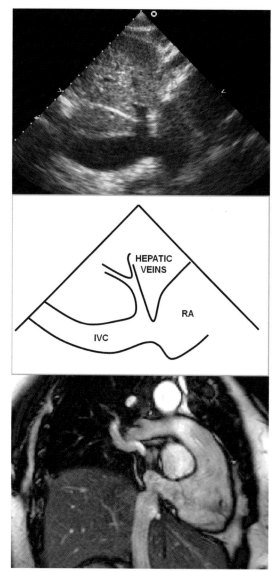

Fig. 2.12 Inferior vena cava imaged by transthoracic echocardiography from a subcostal window (top) and with a specifically positioned oblique sagittal cardiovascular magnetic resonance imaging plane (bottom).

Aortic views

Several imaging planes are used to assess the aorta in both long- and short-axis views.

Names
- Echo—suprasternal view, subcostal aortic view
- TOE—short- and long-axis aortic views from the oesophagus
- CMR—multiple views of aorta possible; standard planes include oblique sagittal view
- CT—multiple views of aorta possible; standard planes include oblique sagittal view
- Nuclear—not often acquired

The view (Fig. 2.13)
The optimal images are those that clearly demonstrate the walls of the aorta.

What do you see?
Aorta
May see wall thickening, aneurysm, or even gross mobile thrombus and plaque.

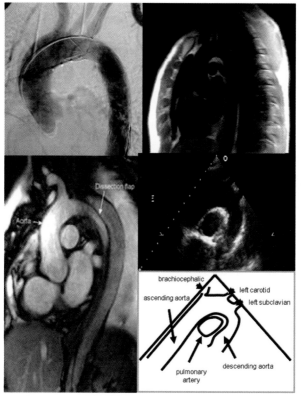

Fig. 2.13 Aortic views. Clockwise from top left: aortography, an oblique sagittal view with cardiovascular magnetic resonance, a suprasternal view with transthoracic echocardiography, and a further cardiovascular magnetic resonance image using a different sequence.

Pulmonary vein views

Pulmonary vein views are important for assessment of anatomy and left atrial inflow.

Names
- Echo—apical four-chamber view (pulmonary veins seen in far distance)
- TOE—different views are needed to image each pulmonary vein.
- CMR—specialized pulmonary vein assessment is obtained from a pulmonary angiogram
- CT—specialized pulmonary vein assessment is obtained from a pulmonary angiogram
- Nuclear—not often acquired

The view (Fig. 2.14)
The optimal views provide information on pulmonary vein anatomy and alignment for flow measures in echocardiography.

Coronary sinus views

Seeing the coronary sinus can be useful in some procedures such as electrophysiology studies or pacing device placement. It also allows assessment of congenital abnormalities such as a persistent left superior vena cava.

Names
- Echo—coronary sinus view
- CMR—coronary sinus view
- CT—coronary sinus view
- Nuclear—not often acquired

The view
The optimal views provide information on the anatomy of the coronary sinus as it wraps around the mitral annulus and enters the right atrium.

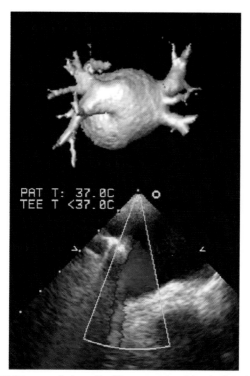

Fig. 2.14 Pulmonary vein views with a 3D reconstruction of the veins derived from gadolinium contrast and cardiovascular magnetic resonance imaging (top), and individual Doppler flow assessment with transoesophageal echocardiography (bottom).

Polar view

This view summarizes all the information from the left ventricular myocardium. Therefore this view is created in post-processing and is most useful for assessment of regional myocardial perfusion defects or changes in myocardial function based on variation in strain patterns.

Names
- Echo—polar view sometimes generated from 3D volume datasets or in stress studies
- TOE—not often acquired
- CMR—not often acquired
- CT—not often acquired
- Nuclear—often presented to demonstrate variation in perfusion

The view (Fig. 2.15)
A map of the left ventricle with the apex in the centre and each wall spreading out to the periphery.

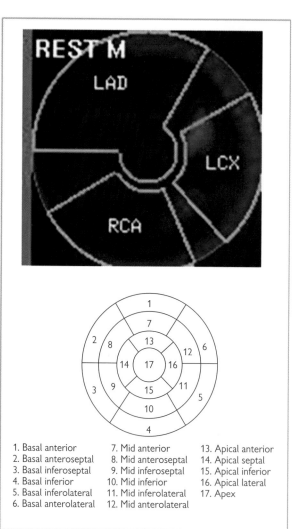

1. Basal anterior
2. Basal anteroseptal
3. Basal inferoseptal
4. Basal inferior
5. Basal inferolateral
6. Basal anterolateral
7. Mid anterior
8. Mid anteroseptal
9. Mid inferoseptal
10. Mid inferior
11. Mid inferolateral
12. Mid anterolateral
13. Apical anterior
14. Apical septal
15. Apical inferior
16. Apical lateral
17. Apex

Fig. 2.15 A polar view of the left ventricle demonstrating myocardial perfusion assessed by nuclear cardiology. Diagram reproduced with permission from Sabharwal N, Loong CY, and Kelion A (2008) *Nuclear Cardiology*, Oxford University Press.

3D reconstructions

3D reconstructions are increasingly being generated from 3D volume datasets. Typically these involve surface rendering that can be adjusted to maximize delineation of cardiac anatomy. They are particularly useful for assessing overall left ventricular shape and valvular function. They are also an integral part of vascular imaging.

Names
- Echo—usually for assessment of LV
- TOE—usually for assessment of valves, in particular the mitral valve, but also for monitoring procedures
- CMR—usually used for venography and angiography
- CT—usually used to provide an overview of the anatomy of coronary vessels
- Nuclear—not usually acquired.

The view (Fig. 2.16)
Because 3D rendering is usually performed after data acquisition the area of interest and view can be tailored to suit the clinical question. The view can also usually be rotated and manipulated to maximize 3D handling.

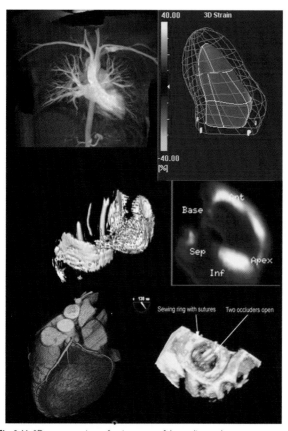

Fig. 2.16 3D reconstructions of various parts of the cardiovascular system.
The aorta (top left) and carotids (middle left) are seen with cardiovascular magnetic
resonance. The surface of the heart and epicardial coronaries (bottom left) are seen
with cardiac CT. The function of the left ventricle is derived from echocardiographic
(top right) and nuclear perfusion (middle right) data. The bottom right shows a 3D
transoesophageal image of a prosthetic mitral valve.

Left ventricular function

Left ventricle 98
Left ventricular function 100
Chest X-ray 104
Echocardiography 106
Cardiac magnetic resonance 112
Radionuclide ventriculography (RNV) 114
Single-photon emission computed tomography (SPECT) 116
Positron emission tomography (PET) 118
Cardiac CT 120
Angiography 122

Left ventricle

Left ventricular deterioration is an important marker of worsening clinical prognosis. Parameters of left ventricular function, generally systolic ejection fraction (EF), are commonly measured in patients with heart disease. The lower the resting EF or the more global the left ventricular dysfunction, the worse the survival. Therefore left ventricular assessment is one of the most frequent indications for cardiovascular imaging.

Anatomy

The left ventricle is an ellipsoid-shaped cavity with muscular walls. It contains the papillary muscles (anterolateral and posteromedial) and chordal attachments to both leaflets of the mitral valve.

Cardiovascular imaging

Invasive cardiac catheterization was the first reliable cardiac imaging technique. Now all non-invasive imaging techniques are able to perform some form of left ventricular assessment. However, there are significant differences in the accuracy and reproducibility of the methods. Optimal use of available techniques is crucial for diagnosis, treatment, and follow-up of patients. The optimal imaging technique needs to be able to measure left ventricular size and mass and also how those measures vary during the cardiac cycle (both systole and diastole). In principle echocardiography provides readily available evaluation of the left ventricle to determine systolic and diastolic function through a combination of 2D and Doppler imaging. However, it may be limited by image quality and CMR provides a far more precise measure of cavity size to determine systolic function although it is limited in its ability to assess diastolic function. Nuclear techniques have been available as a gold standard measure of left ventricular systolic function for many years.

The modalities most often used for left ventricular assessment are:
- Echocardiography.
  - 2D
  - contrast 2D
  - real-time three-dimensional (RT3DE)
  - contrast RT3DE
  - transoesophageal echocardiography (TOE)
- Nuclear imaging.
  - radionuclide ventriculography (RNV)
  - gated SPECT
- Cardiac magnetic resonance (CMR)
- Angiography.

Modalites used less often for left ventricular assessment are:
- Computed tomography (CT)
- Positron emission tomography (PET).

Left ventricular function

Global left ventricular function

Quantitative measurements of left ventricular function have the highest value for the clinical assessment of cardiovascular prognosis. However, imaging modalities vary significantly in their ability to provide accurate and reproducible measurements. This ability depends greatly on the mode of acquisition, which determines the type and accuracy of the geometric assumptions used to reconstruct the heart structure and calculate the cardiac volumes.

Cardiac volumes

Simpson's rule is generally used to determine LV volume. It is based on the principle of slicing the LV from the apex to the mitral valve annulus in a series of discs. The volume of each disc is measured and the volumes summed to give the full volume.

Ejection fraction

Left ventricular systolic function is usually assessed using the ejection fraction (EF) which is expressed as the ratio of stroke volume (SV) to end-diastolic volume (EDV):

$$EF = (SV/EDV) \times 100$$

where SV = EDV − ESV and ESV is the end-systolic volume (Fig. 3.1).
   Although ejection fraction is used it can vary with:
- afterload
- preload
- myocardial contractility
- synchrony of the regional contractile pattern
- heart rate.

Quantitative assessment of systolic function

Quantitative assessment of the LV systolic function is usually based on ejection fraction measurements:

normal systolic function	EF >55%
mild systolic dysfunction	EF 54–45%
moderate systolic dysfunction	EF 44–36%
severe systolic dysfunction	EF <35%

Qualitative assessment of systolic function

Qualitative global cardiac function assessment is often used in a clinical setting. An observer subjectively grades LV function as normal, mild, moderate, or severe systolic dysfunction. This widely used method has acceptable correlations with quantitative assessment, but only for experienced readers.

A – SIMPSON'S RULE

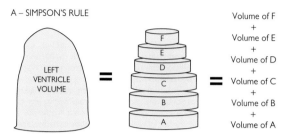

LEFT VENTRICLE VOLUME = (stack of discs F, E, D, C, B, A) =

Volume of F
+
Volume of E
+
Volume of D
+
Volume of C
+
Volume of B
+
Volume of A

SIMPSON'S RULE SIMPLIIFIES THE LEFT VENTRICLE INTO A SERIES OF DISCS WHICH
ARE THEN SUMMED TOGETHER TO CALCULATE THE TOTAL VOLUME.
THE VOLUME OF EACH DISC CAN BE ESTIMATED FROM THE DIAMETER OF THE
VENTRICLE AT EACH LEVEL BASED ON LONG AXIS IMAGING OR A STACK OF SHORT
AXIS IMAGES CAN BE ACQUIRED AND THE AREA AT EACH LEVEL USED TO
ESTIMATE THE DISC VOLUME.

B – EJECTION FRACTION AND STROKE VOLUME

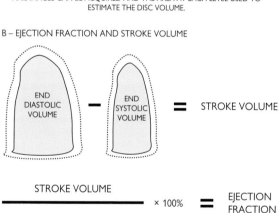

END
DIASTOLIC
VOLUME − END
SYSTOLIC
VOLUME = STROKE VOLUME

$$\frac{\text{STROKE VOLUME}}{\text{END DIASTOLIC VOLUME}} \times 100\% = \text{EJECTION FRACTION}$$

Fig. 3.1 Schematic diagram of the principle of measurement of stroke volume and
ejection fraction.

Regional left ventricular function

Wall motion assessment

Regional wall motion influences global left ventricular function and is an independent predictor of outcome in patients with ischaemic heart disease. However, imaging modalities differ significantly in relation to their ability to recognize wall motion abnormalities.

Unfortunately, at present there are no widely used objective quantitative methods to assess regional wall motion abnormalities in any of the imaging methods. Subjective visual grading is the most frequently used approach. Accurate visual grading of regional wall motion, technically one of the simplest aspects of cardiovascular imaging, is actually one of the most complex and difficult tasks for a cardiovascular imager to learn.

Cardiac segment grading

Cardiac segments are graded as follows.
- **Normal or hyperkinetic**—the LV contour moves concentrically, visible endocardial excursion, normal wall thickening.
- **Hypokinetic**—reduced wall motion and wall thickening.
- **Akinetic**—lack of both motion and wall thickening.
- **Dyskinetic**—outward movement during systole, systolic ventricular wall bulging.
- **Aneurysmal**—thinned ventricular wall.

Models containing 17 segments (most modalities) or 16 segments (echocardiography only, according to the American Society of Echocardiography (ASE) guidelines) are usually used for cardiac wall motion assessment (Fig. 3.2). Factors influencing accuracy of wall motion assessment are:
- image quality
- improper alignment of the imaging planes
- cardiac movement
  - complexity of LV motion—translational motion of the heart and the descent of the aortic and mitral rings
  - tachycardia
  - bundle branch blocks
  - arrhythmias
  - cardiac translational movement.

Diastolic function

Diastolic dysfunction is an important feature of cardiac dysfunction that has proved hard to diagnose or quantify accurately. The basis of diastolic dysfunction is a disorder of relaxation of the myocardium during diastole that leads to inefficient filling of the ventricle. Therefore imaging diastolic function requires an ability to measure movement of the myocardium during diastole or a method of estimating filling of the ventricle.

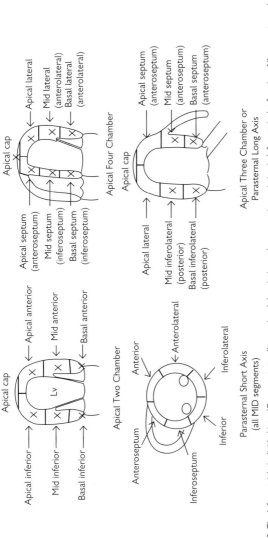

Fig. 3.2 The left ventricle is divided into 17 segments to allow regional descriptions when reporting variation in left ventricular function. All segments can be assessed using the standard imaging planes, and some segments are seen in multiple planes.

Chest X-ray

The chest X-ray (Fig. 3.3) has long been the first line assessment of cardiac function. Often the referral for further cardiovascular imaging is based on the conclusions drawn from clinical skills and the chest X-ray.

Advantages of the chest X-ray
- Widely available
- Image of heart and chest in the same view to allow investigation of differential diagnoses.

Disadvantages of the chest X-ray
- Single view without detailed anatomy or information over the cardiac cycle
- Ionizing radiation.

What does the chest X-ray tell us?
The key signs of interest in the chest X-ray to assess cardiac structure and function are:
- size of cardiac silhouette relative to size of thorax—enlarged heart consistent with cardiac enlargement due to heart failure, hypertrophy, or pericardial fluid
- evidence of fluid in the lungs (e.g. upper lobe blood diversion, fluid in fissures, Kerley B lines).

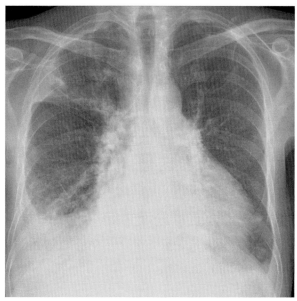

Fig. 3.3 PA chest X-ray. This patient has an increased cardiothoracic ratio suggesting that there may be some form of cardiac pathology such as left ventricular dysfunction, hypertrophy, or pericardial disease.

Echocardiography

Cardiac ultrasound has high spatial resolution and excellent temporal resolution to define left ventricular function, cardiac regional wall thickening, and inward endocardial excursion. Well-established technological advances, such as harmonic imaging and contrast echocardiography, improve image quality in patients with difficult acoustic windows.

Advantages of echocardiography

- High spatial resolution
- High temporal resolution
- Additional structural and physiological information (cardiac, extra-cardiac)
- No ionizing radiation or contrast material needed (but ultrasound contrast agents can be used if required to improve image quality)
- Versatile, widely available, portable, and low cost
- Tissue Doppler and strain analysis allow measures of diastolic function.

Disadvantages of echocardiography

- Poor acoustic windows in some patients
- Through-plane motion of the myocardium in 2D
- High operator dependence
- Better reproducibility is achieved with other imaging modalities that are less operator dependent
- Lack of quantitative ejection fraction—there is no fully reproducible quantitative technique to measure LVEF
- Comparison with angiography and CMR echocardiography may underestimate LV volumes:

Apical Four Chamber

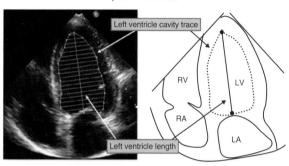

Apical Two Chamber

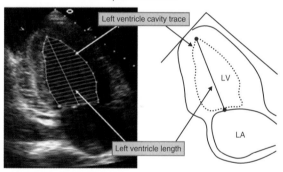

Fig. 3.4 Left ventricular dimensions and ejection fraction can be calculated from 2D imaging. Ideally, biplane images provide more accuracy and 3D images the most precise estimates of volume.

What does echocardiography tell us?

Assessment of appearance, size, and function of left ventricle (Table 3.1)

- Obvious structural changes—abnormal ventricular shape, aneurysms, wall thinning, hypertrophy.
- Quantitative measures of size—normal, mild, moderate, severe dilatation/hypertrophy.
- Appearance—eccentric, concentric, asymmetric, septal, apical hypertrophy.
- M-mode measures in parasternal views are widely used. However, they are very dependent on alignment and take no account of left ventricular shape or regional wall motion abnormalities. 2D measures are less dependent on alignment.
- Quantitative assessment of systolic function (EF) and summary as normal systolic function or as mild, moderate, or severe systolic dysfunction.
- Diastolic function can be assessed simultaneously from mitral valve inflow and tissue Doppler imaging (TDI).
- Other pathologies which relate to the function of left ventricle (valve disease, pericardial, and aortic abnormalities) can be seen and reported.

Views to assess left ventricular function

Each standard view provides information on the left ventricle (Fig. 3.4).

- **Parasternal long axis**—the basal and mid-segments of the septum and posterior wall are visible. This view is used for measurements of wall thickness, LV outflow tract, and LV cavity dimensions.
- **Parasternal short axis**—by angling the probe back and forth, the whole of the LV can be scanned in cross section. The mid-ventricle (mid-papillary) level is used for linear and area measures of LV walls and cavity. Regional wall motion abnormalities can also be assessed: septum, anterior, lateral, and inferior walls (in clockwise order).
- **Apical four-chamber**—provides best views of apex, septum (on left), and lateral wall (on right) for regional assessment. Suitable for tracing ventricular area in end-diastole and end-systole for EF quantitation.
- **Apical two-chamber**—views of inferior (left) and anterior (right) walls.
- **Apical three-chamber**—views of posterior wall (left) and septum (right).

Table 3.1 Assessment of left ventricular function

Global systolic function

- Subjective evaluation of size, shape, regional and global function
- Measurement of left ventricular volumes/dimensions, ejection fractions (Simpson's rule)
- Doppler—volumetric measurements, dP/dt in patients with mitral regurgitation
- New techniques for myocardial function (strain, strain rate)
- Left ventricular response to exercise test

Left ventricular shape and wall stress

Regional systolic function

- Subjective evaluation of segmental function, wall motion score
- Myocardial contrast enhancement

Diastolic function

- Transmitral flow categorization
- Strategies for recognition of pseudonormal filling
- Left atrial size (area or volume)
- Annular tissue Doppler (E/E')
- Response to Valsalva manoeuvre
- Others (pulmonary vein flow, mitral flow propagation)

Synchrony

- M-mode intraventricular delay
- Doppler assessment of intraventricular delay
- Tissue Doppler imaging

Reproduced with permission from Leeson P, Mitchell A, and Becher (2007) *Echocardiography*, Oxford University Press.

3D echocardiography (Fig. 3.5)

RT3DE is more accurate than 2D echocardiography because it relies less on geometric models. There is also good correlation of the volume measurements with angiographic and CMR data.

Limitations of RT3DE

- Lower spatial and temporal resolution compared with 2D echocardiography
- Artefacts related to:
  - changes in cardiac cycle and respiration
  - motion of the transducer
  - stitching of subvolumes in the full-volume acquisition mode.

Transoesophageal echocardiography

TOE is especially useful for:

- acutely ill patients in intensive care
- patients after cardiothoracic surgery without accessibility to the pre-cordial region for a routine transthoracic echocardiogram

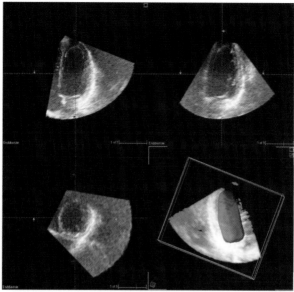

Fig. 3.5 Newer technologies in echocardiography are being developed to improve 3D image quality and further increase the accuracy of left ventricular assessment.

Cardiac magnetic resonance

Cardiac magnetic resonance (CMR) is based on detection of the oscillation of hydrogen atoms in magnetic field to visualize the heart. A scanner acquires multiple slices covering the volume containing the heart and allowing further post-processing of the image. High image quality translates into outstanding reproducibility. Therefore CMR is able to detect discrete changes in LV volume and mass in individual patients. It is considered the gold standard for assessment of cardiac volume and cardiac mass.

Advantages of CMR

- Absence of ionizing radiation.
- High-resolution anatomical detail.
- Unique combination of anatomy, function, blood flow, and myocardial tissue characterization of the heart.
- Accurate measurements of wall thickness and LV mass—applicable to serial assessment monitoring interventions on LV remodelling.
- Accurate assessment of regional and global LV function.
- Ability to assess pericardial/extracardial structures.

Disadvantages of CMR

- Currently slow acquisition with multiple breathholds.
- Need for meticulous cardiac and respiratory gating/breathholding.
- Most of current designs are unsuitable for claustrophobic patients.
- Need for correction for cardiac and respiratory motion.
- If paramagnetic contrast agents (gadolinium-based) are necessary, contraindications apply.
- Patients with metallic objects, pacemakers, and other devices are excluded.
- High equipment cost.

What does CMR tell us?

CMR has important advantages for left ventricular imaging because of its superior image quality and lack of radiation. CMR represents a gold standard approach for assessment of left ventricular volumes during the cardiac cycle and therefore can provide a precise assessment of ejection fraction (Fig. 3.6).

Advanced techniques such as CMR tagging involve labelling a specific segment of myocardium by application of tags, which move and deform with the myocardium. This method provides the capability to quantify transmural myocardial excursion, wall thickening, circumferential shortening, and longitudinal shortening simultaneously. Although it is mostly used in the research setting at present, CMR offers a unique method for quantifying regional wall motion during systole.

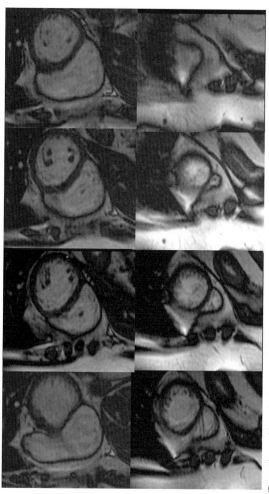

Fig. 3.6 CMR provides a gold standard assessment of left ventricular size because it is possible to collect multiple short axis planes down the length of the left ventricle. Volumes in each plane can be summed (equivalent to Simpson's method) to model the left ventricle accurately.

Radionuclide ventriculography (RNV)

Simple planar scintigraphic imaging, like radionuclide ventriculography (RNV) (alternative names refer to different methods of acquiring images: equilibrium radionuclide ventriculography (ERNV), radionuclide angiography (RNA), radionuclide cine angiography (RNCA), multiple-gated cardiac blood pool imaging (MUGA), equilibrium radionuclide angio-graphy (ERNA), first-pass radionuclide angiography (FPRNA)) was the first widely used non-invasive method for quantification of left ventricular function. It involves radionuclide labelling of the patient's blood pool with a radio-active tracer (usually *in vivo*, but sometimes *in vitro*) and summing ECG-gated counts from successive cardiac cycles over several minutes (Fig. 3.7). Radioactivity is measured by a gamma camera over the anterior chest. The radionuclide most frequently used is technetium-99m (^{99m}Tc). Left anterior oblique (LAO) and left posterior oblique (LPO) projections are usually used for acquisition. The number of counts recorded is proportional to the amount of the blood radioactivity, which is linearly related to the blood volume.

Advantages of radionuclide ventriculography

- High accuracy.
- High reproducibility with low inter- and intra-observer variability (usually <5%).
- Measurements do not depend on the geometry of the left ventricle.
- Technically easy to perform with little dependence on the operator (but, like all methods, it is still dependent on reporting experience).
- Appropriate for serial monitoring of LV ejection fraction measurements (e.g. in patients receiving cardiotoxic chemotherapy).
- Extensive literature showing its prognostic value and cost-effectiveness.

Disadvantages of radionuclide ventriculography

- Radiation exposure.
- Low spatial resolution which limits anatomical characterization of the structures.
- Regional wall motion can be assessed, but not regional systolic thickening of the myocardium.
- Ancillary anatomical information is not obtained (e.g. presence of thrombi, valve dysfunction, diseases of the pericardium).

What does radionuclide ventriculography tell us?

Count-based quantitative EF measurements are highly accurate and independent of LV shape. It is not necessary to calculate LV volumes to obtain EF values. It has excellent correlation with cardiac catheterization contrast ventriculography and CMR.

This technique can be used for virtually all patients, if they have no contraindications for nuclear imaging.

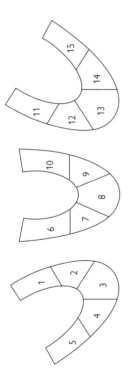

Anterior	LAO	Left lateral
1. Basal anterolateral	6. Septal	11. Basal anterior
2. Mid anterolateral	7. Inferoseptal	12. Mid anterior
3. Apical	8. Inferoapical	13. Apex
4. Mid inferoseptal	9. Inferolateral	14. Mid inferior
5. Basal inferoseptal	10. Lateral	15. Basal inferior

Fig. 3.7 In nuclear cardiology blood pool imaging allows accurate quantification of left ventricular function. Gated imaging also allows assessment of regional variation, and the different segments of the left ventricle can be viewed from the planar imaging segments. Reproduced with permission from Sabharwal N, Loong CY and Kelion A (2008) *Nuclear Cardiology*, Oxford University Press.

Single-photon emission computed tomography (SPECT)

Simple planar scintigraphic imaging has generally been replaced by imaging more relevant for cardiac applications—radionuclide myocardial perfusion scintigraphy. SPECT is based on the flow-dependent selective uptake of a radioactive tracer by functional myocardial tissue. Myocardial perfusion scintigraphy SPECT is acquired as a series of planar projections from different angles of the gamma camera circulating the patient. A reconstruction method is then used to receive standard sections through the heart with enhanced image quality. Currently most centres use SPECT gated to the ECG to obtain slices at a particular point of the cardiac cycle. This is known as gated SPECT (Fig 3.8) and allows assessment of perfusion. However, information on cardiac motion and size can also be obtained.

Advantages of SPECT

- Global LV ejection fraction and LV volumes are measured accurately and reproducibly.
- Relatively operator independent for data acquisition (but like all methods still dependent on reporting experience).
- Applicable to most referred patients, including:
  - obese patients not suitable for echocardiography ('difficult echo windows')
  - claustrophobic patients who cannot tolerate MR or CT
  - patients with implanted devices not suitable for MR (heating, displacement) or CT (artefacts).
- Assessment of systolic thickening and wall motion.
- Simultaneous evaluation of perfusion and function.
- Viability assessment.
- Improved ability to risk stratify patients by providing information relevant to the global LVEF.
- Extensive literature showing its prognostic value and cost-effectiveness.
- Cost-effective and suitable for high-volume service.

Disadvantages of SPECT

- Radiation exposure.
- Low spatial resolution—lower spatial resolution than ultrasonography and especially CMR.
- Artefacts caused by partial volume effects.
- No ancillary structural information obtained.
- Decreased accuracy of LVEF assessment with large perfusion defects.
- Lack of portability.

What does SPECT tell us?

Visual grading of LV global and regional function based on gated SPECT images has been shown to correlate favourably with visual grading by CMR. Automated determination of the LVEF, and thus a quantitative global EF and percentage of thickening in various regions, can be used. Gated SPECT underestimates the ejection fraction when compared with equilibrium radionuclide angiography in patients with LV dysfunction and large perfusion defects.

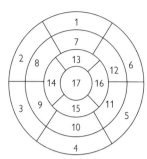

1. Basal anterior
2. Basal anteroseptal
3. Basal inferoseptal
4. Basal inferior
5. Basal inferolateral
6. Basal anterolateral

7. Mid anterior
8. Mid anteroseptal
9. Mid inferoseptal
10. Mid inferior
11. Mid inferolateral
12. Mid anterolateral

13. Apical anterior
14. Apical septal
15. Apical inferior
16. Apical lateral
17. Apex

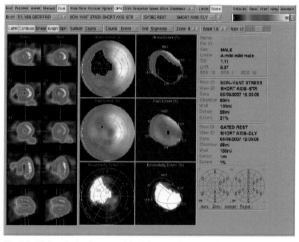

Fig. 3.8 (A) Standard polar view of the left ventricle used in nuclear imaging with the different regions of the ventricle annotated. (B) An example of quantitative analysis of a reversible antero-apical and septal perfusion defect. Reproduced with permission from Sabharwal N, Loong CY and Kelion A (2008) *Nuclear Cardiology*, Oxford University Press.

Positron emission tomography (PET)

This is only a brief presentation of the method, which is highly specialized and is available only in a limited number of centres. It uses radiopharmaceuticals producing pairs of photons imaged by special gamma cameras.

If fluorine-18 fluorodeoxyglucose (FDG) metabolic tracer is used, PET is the most sensitive technique for myocardial viability. Additionally, it can measure global LV function and evaluate regional wall motion.

Radionuclides used most frequently
- Rubidium-82 (^{82}Rb).
- Nitrogen-13 ammonia (^{13}N-ammonia).
- Fluorine-18 fluorodeoxyglucose (^{18}F-FDG).

Advantages of PET
- Superior quality to SPECT, resulting in higher diagnostic accuracy.
- Unique metabolic technique for myocardial viability.

Disadvantages of PET
- Radiation exposure.
- Very limited availability with expensive set-up of special gamma camera–cyclotron–radiochemistry facility.

Cardiac CT

Computed tomography (CT) is based on the principle that fan-shaped thin X-ray beams pass through body at many angles and enter the detector array to create cross-sectional images.

New CT techniques, such as electron-beam CT (EBCT) and especially multidetector CT (MDCT), have significantly reduced the time required for image acquisition and improved image quality. MDCT allows very fast acquisition of a cardiac dataset with a very good spatial resolution and signal intensity, allowing extensive post-processing of the image.

Advantages of Cardiac CT

- High speed of acquisition—within one breathhold.
- High spatial resolution.
- Good reproducibility.
- Very good endocardial delineation (with contrast).
- Ancillary cardiac/extracardiac anatomical information.
- Applicable for patients with cardiac devices needing a high-resolution imaging test.
- Image post-processing in long and short axis and 3D reconstruction.

Disadvantages of cardiac CT

- Radiation exposure (although exposure is significantly decreased in newly developed techniques).
- Intravenous contrast has to be used to separate the myocardium from the blood pool but it can be the same injection as for the coronary arteries.
- Additional sets of cardiac images at end-diastole and end-systole increase radiation exposure.
- Currently limited mostly to anatomical rather than functional information (Fig. 3.9).
- Quantitative aspects limited if there are significant arrhythmias (e.g. atrial fibrillation).

What does cardiac CT tell us?

Left ventricular function assessment is not a routine indication for a cardiac CT. Nevertheless, ejection fraction can be measured concomitantly in patients referred for CT coronary angiography and therefore can add to its clinical value as part of the test.

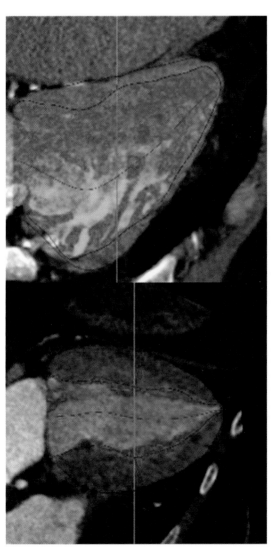

Fig. 3.9 Left ventricular size can be measured with cardiac CT based on techniques that rely on variations in attenuation to identify left ventricular boundaries.

Angiography

Angiography was the first established imaging technique used for highly reproducible left ventricular assessment (Fig. 3.10). It is still often used as the gold standard with which non-invasive techniques have been compared. Absolute volumes are highly reproducible and are often recommended as yielding the most precise quantitative measurements of global function of all the imaging techniques. LV volumes can be calculated using the area–length method, which uses modelling of the cardiac chambers based on the area and length of the left ventricle (area–length formula). Biplane assessment is recommended over single plane, and Simpson's rule can be applied. Biplane angiography is used in 25° RAO and 80° LAO projections. The total volume is calculated as the sum of the volumes of the individual segments.

Advantages of angiography

- Simultaneous measurements of intracavitary pressures and other haemodynamic variables.
- Concomitant cardiac diagnoses.
- Associated valvular lesions such as mitral or aortic regurgitation simultaneously diagnosed and semi-quantitated.
- Left-to-right shunts at the atrial and ventricular levels.
- Coronary angiography and coronary interventions during the same cardiac catherization procedure.

Disadvantages of angiography

- Invasive nature.
- Radiation exposure.
- Potential nephrotoxicity of the dye.
- LV mass and hypertrophy are better quantitated by echocardiography and especially CMR.
- Abnormal wall motion, but not abnormal thickening, can be assessed by ventriculography.
- High cost.

What does left ventriculography tell us?

Angiography provides a precise chamber area although it has a tendency to overestimate LV volumes. Therefore regression equations can be used. Left and right haemodynamic measures can provide assessments of diastolic as well as systolic function.

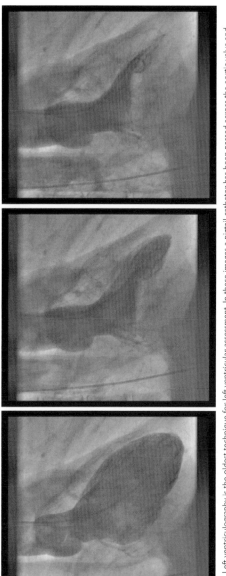

Fig. 3.10 Left ventriculography is the oldest technique for left ventricular assessment. In these images a pigtail catheter has been passed across the aortic valve and positioned within the left ventricle. Dye is then injected at a fixed rate and fluoroscopy performed to capture images of the left ventricle throughout the cardiac cycle. Reproduced with permission from Mitchell ARJ, West NEJ, Leeson P, and Banning AP (2008) Cardiac Catheterization and Coronary Intervention, Oxford University Press.

Myocardium

Myocardial imaging *126*
Echocardiography *128*
Cardiac magnetic resonance *132*
Cardiac CT *136*
Coronary angiography *136*

Myocardial imaging

Imaging the ventricular myocardium is of critical importance for identifying patients with changes in myocardial size and mass. Further evaluation is required to understand why a particular patient may have changes in (1) myocardial shape or size and (2) myocardial function. The available imaging techniques can be divided into two groups.

The majority of techniques image the myocardial tissue directly:
• echocardiography (transthoracic 2D)
• CMR
• CT.

Other modalities image the myocardial tissue indirectly:
• Nuclear cardiology

Contrast and other injected agents

Contrast or other injected agents are usually used to optimize assessment of the myocardium. These increase the visibility of the myocardium, the blood flow through the tissue, and the metabolism within the tissue.

Injected agents can have the following properties.
• They flow through the microvessels (microbubbles, ultrasound contrast—myocardial contrast echocardiography (MCE)).
• They flow through the epicardial vessels and microcirculation (iodinated contrast agents—cardiac CT).
• They flow through the microvessels and leak into the myocardium (gadolinium contrast agents—CMR).
• They bind to the myocardium (radioactive tracers—nuclear cardiology).
• They are used within myocardial metabolism (radioactive tracers—PET).

Agents are chosen because their unique properties mean that they provide a signal that can easily be identified by the imaging modality. The resolution of the imaging in this situation depends on the size of the agent used or, if the agent attaches to a particular cellular target, the size of that target.

Molecular imaging

Agents may become available that combine an agent easily seen with a particular imaging modality with a receptor or antibody that binds to a specific molecular target within the myocardium. This could be used to measure change in, for example, aspects of inflammation or ischaemia.

Increased myocardial size

Possible causes of increased myocardial size or thickness include:

- hypertensive heart disease
- infiltrative cardiomyopathies
- hypertrophic cardiomyopathies
- cardiac tumours.

All these diseases can also lead to changes in function, typically evidence of diastolic dysfunction or a restrictive cardiomyopathy.

Masses in the heart

Cardiovascular imaging is essential in the identification and characterization of cardiac tumours. Echocardiography is usually the first modality to identify the mass and then further imaging with cardiovascular magnetic resonance of cardiac CT provides detailed assessment of position of mass, tissue characteristics and extent size.

Masses in the heart include:

Primary tumours (benign)

- myoxma
- papillary fibroelastoma
- lipoma
- fibroma
- rhabdomyoma.

Primary tumours (malignant)

- sarcomas
- angiosarcomas
- rhabdomyosarcomas
- primary lymphoma.

Secondary tumours

- metastases.

Cysts

Extra cardiac tumours

Echocardiography

Echocardiography is the most commonly used first-line investigational technique to assess the myocardium. Echocardiography provides assessment of:

- left ventricular size on standard 2D second-harmonic echocardiography
- myocardial function by Doppler imaging.

Both may be observer dependent, and echocardiogrpahy has limited ability to dissect out differential diagnoses. Therefore more detailed imaging, typically with cardiovascular magnetic resonance, is usually warranted once echocardiography has identified myocardial disease.

Cardiac masses

Echocardiography provides immediate identification of presence, appearance, and location of a cardiac mass. This may be enough to identify the likely nature of the mass, e.g. atrial myxoma is often attached to septum and has cystic elements. Echocardiography is particularly good at identifying cystic structures as the fluid filled centre appears dark.

Ultrasound contrast will be evident in any microvessels in the mass. If the mass remains dark then it is likely to represent thrombus or be cystic.

Left ventricular hypertrophy

The simplest thing to observe with echocardiography is a change in the size of the heart muscle. Echocardiographic assessment of left ventricular hypertrophy is more accurate and reproducible than ECG-based criteria.

- Estimation of left ventricular mass can be undertaken based on measures in several views. Mass assessment is usually limited by the image quality of the endocardial border.
- Wall thickness is often assessed, and regional variation in thickness can usually be assessed qualitatively.

Hypertrophic cardiomyopathy

Echocardiography may be diagnostic for hypertrophic cardiomyopathy.

- It can identify increased left ventricular mass and wall thickening.
- It can identify regional asymmetric variation (typically asymmetric septal hypertrophy but sometimes apical hypertrophy) (Fig. 4.1).
- It can identify a hyperdynamic ejection fraction with cavity obliteration.
- Doppler and M-mode can demonstrate left ventricular outflow obstruction related to septal hypertrophy.

Cardiac amyloid

- Cardiac amyloid is suggested by the presence of echocardiographic-derived ventricular hypertrophy in the presence of small-amplitude complexes on ECG (Fig. 4.2).
- The presence of valvular and atrial wall thickening may also be seen.
- Increased 'speckling' within the myocardium can also sometimes be seen, although this is a less reliable sign as it is dependent on ultrasound gain settings.

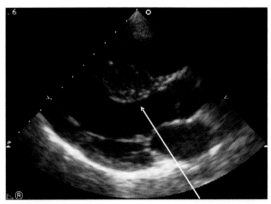

Fig. 4.1 Parasternal long-axis transthoracic echocardiography view. The patient has hypertrophic cardiomyopathy which is evident from the asymmetric septal hyptrophy (arrow).

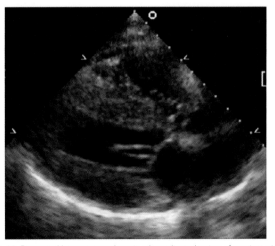

Fig. 4.2 Parasternal long-axis transthoracic echocardiography view of a patient with cardiac amyloid. Note the global gross hypertrophy and bright speckled appearance of the myocardium.

Other infiltrative cardiomyopathies

Other infiltrative diseases (e.g. sarcoid, endomyocardial fibrosis, and haemochromatosis) may produce similar ventricular hypertrophy. However, they do not have specific signs on echocardiography and the modality cannot be relied upon to diagnose infiltrative disease.

Left ventricular non-compaction

This specific abnormality of increased trabeculation of the left ventricular wall can be identified on echocardiography and the appearances are enhanced by the use of left ventricular contrast agents that highlight the trabeculations (Fig. 4.3).

Doppler

A key aspect of myocardial assessment with echocardiography in a patient with changes in myocardial size or function is the use of tissue Doppler to assess myocardial motion. This can be combined with a pulse-wave Doppler signal from the mitral valve inflow to understand the relation between ventricular filling and ventricular motion. This information allows investigation of:
- diastolic heart failure
- restrictive cardiomyopathy versus constrictive physiology
- regional wall motion abnormalities
- dyssynchrony.

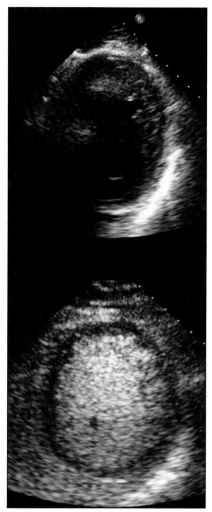

Fig. 4.3 Transthoracic echocardiography in a short-axis view before (top) and after (bottom) left ventricular contrast. The patient has left ventricular non-compaction and there is evidence of increased trabeculation of the lateral wall of the left ventricle.

Cardiac magnetic resonance

CMR is undoubtedly the best imaging modality for directly assessing the characteristics of tissue within the myocardium. It provides information on the following.
- Left and right ventricular mass.
- Left and right ventricular volumes and ejection fractions.
- Left and right ventricular wall thickening/motion.
- Late gadolinium enhancement can help to differentiate between ischaemic and non-ischaemic cardiomyopathy (dilated cardiomyopathy).
- Patterns of late gadolinium enhancement can be used to guide diagnosis and prognosis in some conditions.
- Features of restrictive filling such as abnormal septal motion, atrial enlargement, and abnormal IVC appearances (Fig. 4.4).
- Exclusion of other causes of symptoms such as pericardial thickening or disease.
- Serial monitoring of changes in the myocardium.

Cardiac masses

The advantages of CMR are that the multiple imaging planes allow easy characterization of size and extent of any cardiac mass. Involvement of extra cardiac structures can be assessed. The tissue characteristics of the mass can also be demonstrated using different sequences and it is possible to see whether it perfuses using contrast e.g. no perfusion is seen in thrombus.

Left ventricular hypertrophy

CMR provides a means for precise assessment of left ventricular mass. However, it is not usually required for patients with left ventricular hypertrophy related to hypertension as it does not provide significant additional information. The main indication is for those with hypertrophy in whom there is uncertainty about the underlying diagnosis.

Hypertrophic cardiomyopathy

Use of CMR in patients with hypertrophic cardiomyopathy is increasingly becoming the standard pattern of care in view of its ability to confirm diagnosis and provide information using late gadolinium enhancement that may be prognostic. The key features of hypertrophic cardiomyopathy on CMR are:
- increased left (and right) ventricular mass.
- regional variation in mass (typically septal but also apical) with asymmetry.
- hyperdynamic left ventricular function with cavity obliteration.

Contrast images show:
- Late gadolinium enhancement either in the area of hypertrophy to suggest fibrosis or typically at the inferior and/or superior LV–RV junction (Fig. 4.5).

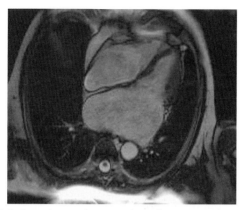

Fig. 4.4 Cardiovascular magnetic resonance images from a patient with a restrictive cardiomyopathy. The most striking feature is the gross bilateral atrial enlargement.

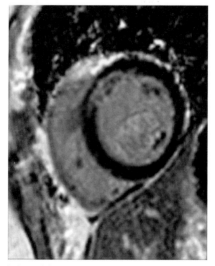

Fig. 4.5 Patchy late gadolinium enhancement on cardiovascular magnetic resonance imaging in the superior part of the septum in a patient being investigated for a cardiomyopathy.

Cardiac amyloid

Cardiac amyloid has distinctive appearances on CMR (Fig. 4.6). Non-contrast images demonstrate:
- global increased left ventricular mass
- often other features of a restrictive cardiomyopathy including bilateral enlargement.

Contrast images show:
- global uptake of gadolinium which persists for a long period of time and is often associated with an unusually dark blood pool.

Other infiltrative cardiomyopathies

Other conditions which can benefit from tissue characterization with CMR include the following.
- Iron overload (e.g. thalassaemia)—the standard image sequence for assessing this is the $T_2{}^*$ image which focuses on the change in T_2 relaxation related to iron deposition in the myocardium
- Other infiltrative cardiomyopathies are usually characterized by diffuse patchy uptake. The patterns may not necessarily be diagnostic except in some conditions where there is known localization such as endomyocardial fibrosis.
- Infiltrative cardiomyopathies can also lead to features of restrictive filling.

Dilated cardiomyopathy

- In dilated cardiomyopathy CMR can demonstrate:
  - increased cardiac volumes
  - thinned myocardium with reduced wall motion.
- Late gadolinium enhancement (LGE)
  - The typical pattern is a thin layer of mid-wall enhancement, often in the lateral wall. Where endocardial regional LGE is seen this is more suggestive of ischaemic aetiology.

Left ventricular non-compaction

Left ventricular non-compaction is easily seen on CMR, and the detailed multiplane imaging allows precise measures of the size of the non-compacted area relative to the compacted myocardium as well as location of the non-compaction.

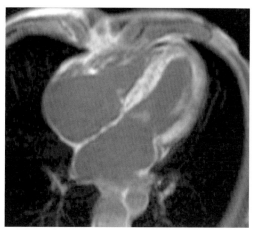

Fig. 4.6 CMR horizontal long-axis view following gadolinium. Note the very bright global changes in the myocardium which also involve the atrial walls. This patient had cardiac amyloid.

Cardiac CT

Gated retrospective acquisitions allow determination of global and regional ventricular function, ejection fraction, and masses, but cardiac CT is not usually a first-line test for myocardial disease.

Possible indications include:
- investigation of pericardial disease to help in diagnosis of the differential between constrictive and restrictive physiology
- non-invasive assessment of coronary anatomy for exclusion of coronary artery disease in dilated and other cardiomyopathies
- investigation of cardiac and extracardiac masses to determine their extent and location.

Coronary angiography

Coronary imaging may be useful in cardiomyopathy patients to exclude an ischaemic (and therefore potentially treatable) aetiology.

Chapter 5

Coronary artery disease

Coronary artery disease *138*
Myocardial ischaemia *140*
Coronary angiogram *144*
Cardiac CT *146*
Cardiac magnetic resonance *148*
Nuclear cardiology *150*
Echocardiography *152*

Coronary artery disease

Non-invasive imaging has become a valuable method for cardiovascular assessment in atherosclerotic coronary artery disease. It plays a crucial role in:
- the initial detection of coronary artery disease
- determining prognosis
- therapeutic decision-making.

A range of techniques using stress protocols are now available to assess myocardial ischaemia or viability in patients with coronary artery disease.

Basic investigations

Careful clinical assessment is an essential prerequisite to the imaging of coronary artery disease (Fig. 5.1). Setting the pre-test probability of a patient having ischaemic heart disease is useful for determining which test is most appropriate, or indeed whether it is appropriate to proceed to non-invasive imaging.

A detailed history for classic symptoms of angina and risk factors, along with a baseline ECG may provide the necessary information to diagnose coronary artery disease. The ECG may also determine which imaging technique is most appropriate and whether there is other unexpected pathology. Baseline blood tests may be important prior to invasive coronary imaging to identify issues such as pre-existing renal dysfunction and anaemia which affect procedural risk and may require investigation before imaging is performed. Assessment of troponin levels is essential in the patient with acute presentation to give a guide to the presence and severity of myocardial infraction.

Cardiovascular imaging

- Direct coronary imaging with angiography may be indicated in patients with stable angina to allow identification of prognostically important coronary disease (such as triple-vessel disease or disease of the left main-stem). Such patients may benefit prognostically from surgical revascularization. Other patients with stable symptoms may undergo invasive coronary imaging with a view to potential revascularization on symptomatic grounds or non invasive coronary imaging with cardiac CT may be appropriate.
- In other situations a functional assessment of the extent of inducible myocardial ischaemia is warranted to provide further information on diagnosis and prognosis without the need for invasive investigation or exposure to ionizing radiation and other risks of angiography.
- Imaging in patients who have had acute coronary events or myocardial infarction is usually performed:
  - to confirm or exclude a clinical diagnosis of atheromatous coronary disease, often as a prerequisite to appropriate revascularization by either percutaneous coronary intervention (PCI) or coronary artery bypass graft (CABG)—echocardiography, coronary angiography
  - to determine the extent of disease and damage to the myocardium and the viability of the myocardium for longer-term management—echocardiography, CMR.

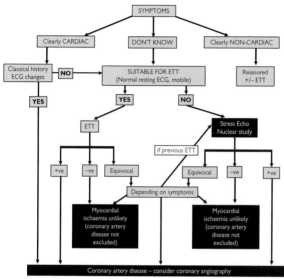

Fig. 5.1 Schematic diagram demonstrating an approach to the management of a patient with suspected coronary artery disease based on symptoms, coronary angiography, and non-invasive imaging. In practice, the choice of non-invasive imaging is largely dependent on local expertise and availability. ETT, exercise tolerance test.

Myocardial ischaemia

The rationale for stress protocols in coronary artery disease is to look for evidence of myocardial ischaemia to aid diagnosis of coronary disease and decide on how to manage the patient i.e. need for revascularization or medical therapy. Ischaemia is identified as a relative reduction in myocardial blood flow on stress sufficient to cause a decrease in myocardial perfusion or contraction. In a normal subject, coronary and myocardial blood flow increases three- to fourfold during stress to match increased myocardial oxygen demand. This can occur because myocardial arteriolar resistance reduces. If there is a coronary stenosis, the arteriolar resistance is already reduced at rest to preserve coronary blood flow. Therefore at rest severe occlusions do not result in wall motion abnormalities, but on stress the blood flow cannot be increased further and the myocardial oxygen delivery is reduced. The more severe the stenosis, the smaller is the possible increase in coronary blood flow and the earlier wall motion abnormalities occur.

Ischaemic cascade: wall motion and perfusion

The ischaemic cascade suggests that perfusion changes occur before regional wall motion abnormalities, which occur before ECG changes, which occur before angina (Fig. 5.2). Therefore techniques which image perfusion may be more sensitive than those relying on regional wall motion abnormalities. In practice the transition through the ischaemic cascade is often quite rapid so that the patient develops perfusion changes, wall motion abnormalities, and angina at a certain 'tipping point' in their stress protocol.

Which technique for ischaemia assessment

Non-invasive imaging techniques have similar sensitivity and specificity for assessment of ischaemia so the choice of test often depends on local availability and expertise. The indications for stress echo-cardiography widely overlap with the indications for myocardial scintigraphy and stress CMR.

There are clinical situations where myocardial scintigraphy is relatively contraindicated (left bundle branch block, bifascicular block, and ventricular paced rhythms). In these situations dynamic exercise leads to perfusion abnormalities of the septum and adjacent walls in the absence of obstructive coronary disease. If there is local expertise, stress echocardiography is an option.

For assessment of viability/hibernation stress echocardiography and myocardial perfusion imaging are joined by MRI and PET. All are potential methods and currently there is no consensus as to whether one of these methods is superior. The decision depends on local availability and expertise.

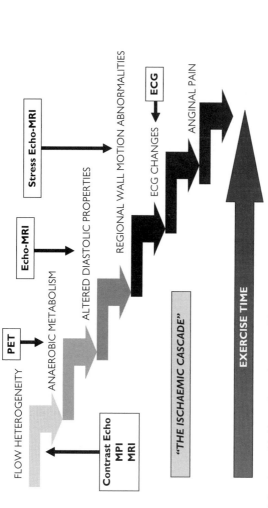

Fig. 5.2 The 'ischaemic cascade' with superimposed imaging modalities positioned to demonstrate the different aspects of developing ischaemia that they are optimized to identify.

Exercise ECG

A normal exercise stress test is useful for the identification of low-risk patients who require no further coronary imaging. However, this test is of little use in those with baseline ECG abnormalities and those who cannot exercise to an adequate level. There is also a significant false-positive rate, especially in women.

Echocardiography

- 2D echocardiography is best suited to assessing regional wall motion abnormalities and therefore is usually used in combination with dobutamine (or exercise) stress.
- Echocardiography allows monitoring of wall motion in real time and the protocol can be ended as the patient develops abnormalities.
- Myocardial contrast echocardiography increasingly offers possibilities for echocardiographic assessment of perfusion simultaneously with wall motion monitoring. This may improve the sensitivity of stress protocols and allow the use of vasodilator stress agents.

Nuclear cardiology

- The basis of nuclear cardiology is the assessment of myocardial perfusion by the radioactive tracer.
- As the pattern of myocardial perfusion that will be identified by the gamma camera is fixed at the point when the tracer is injected, sub-sequent imaging can be performed some time after the stress is complete. Therefore exercise stress is often used with nuclear cardiology.
- Vasodilator stress to maximize changes in perfusion is the next preferred stress modality in those not able to exercise.
- Dobutamine can be used when patients have particular contra-indications to other stress agents.

CMR

- Gadolinium contrast allows the opportunity for imaging of perfusion of the myocardium over a cardiac cycle.
- Therefore CMR tends to be performed with vasodilator stress to maximize changes in perfusion. Regional wall motion abnormalities may be evident at the same time as the perfusion defects.
- CMR can be performed with other stress agents including exercise and dobutamine.

Stress protocols

Exercise stress

Exercise is the most physiological stressor for assessment of myocardial ischaemia in patients able to exercise. It is possible that a treadmill may be advantageous for milder forms of coronary artery disease. Most imaging techniques struggle to obtain good image quality during exercise stress (apart from nuclear techniques in which myocardial imaging can be performed for some time after the exercise is completed).

Dobutamine stress

Dobutamine is given as a graded infusion which increases myocardial oxygen demand in a fashion analogous to staged exercise. Contractility, heart rate, and systolic blood pressure are all increased.

Vasodilators

Vasodilators are effective because they induce regional variation in coronary blood flow. Dipyridamole or adenosine cause a twofold or more increase in myocardial blood flow in segments supplied by normal coronary arteries, whereas flow is unchanged or decreased in segments supplied by stenotic arteries. If oxygen demand increases with flow changes, regional abnormalities in wall motion and thickening appear.

Pacing stress

Exercise, dobutamine, and vasodilator protocols are applicable in most paced patients. Pacing alone only produces chronotropic stress and therefore is usually considered to have a lower sensitivity than pharmacological stress. Patients with a pacemaker cannot undergo CMR.

Coronary angiography

Acute ST-elevation myocardial infarction (STEMI)

Primary PCI

Acute STEMI is the result of thrombotic occlusion of a major epicardial coronary artery. Patient prognosis is dependent on urgent reperfusion of the infarct-related artery. Provided that this can be done in a timely fashion, immediate coronary intervention (primary PCI) is the best method for achieving early reperfusion and long-term outcomes.

Convalescent PCI

In areas without primary PCI initial reperfusion in STEMI is achieved with thrombolysis. Following successful thrombolysis patients may undergo interval angiography and appropriate revascularization. In particular PCI to the infarct-related artery in this context reduces the risk of early reinfarction.

Rescue PCI

This is applied in STEMI patients where thrombolysis has been used but failed to lead to timely reperfusion of the infarct-related artery (lack of ST-segment resolution at 90min). Patients have been shown to benefit from urgent coronary imaging with a view to infarct vessel 'rescue' PCI.

Non-ST-elevation myocardial infarction (NSTEMI)

Patients presenting with acute coronary syndromes (usually characterized by ECG changes other than ST-elevation and/or an elevated plasma troponin level) should be considered for coronary imaging with a view to percutaneous revascularization of the culprit lesion. This early invasive approach has been shown to reduce the risk of future coronary events.

Unstable angina

Patients presenting with a history of rapidly progressive or rest angina may also benefit from coronary imaging and appropriate revascularization.

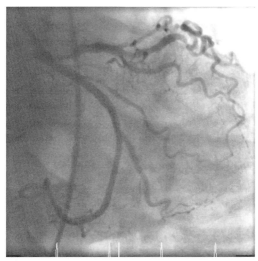

Fig. 5.3 Coronary angiogram. In this projection luminal narrowing is evident in the proximal segment of the left anterior descending artery.

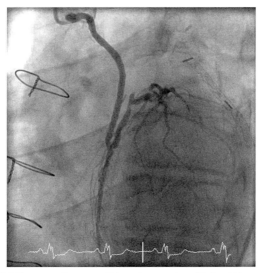

Fig. 5.4 Coronary angiogram on which a saphenous vein graft to the right coronary artery has been intubated. The image demonstrates a patent graft.

Cardiac CT

Non-contrast enhanced cardiac CT and coronary calcium scoring

Non-contrast enhanced cardiac CT is used to identify calcium deposition. Calcium deposition appears "bright white" on CT and can reflect any chronic inflammatory disease process. In coronary disease calcification represents

- In coronaries reflects long standing atherosclerosis and is a marker for increased cardiac events (📖 Coronary calcium scoring p. 48).
- In the myocardium chronic inflammation, most commonly prior to myocardial infarction.

Contrast enhanced cardiac CT and coronary CT

Cardiac CT is an effective way to image coronary arteries and is increasingly used particularly in lower risk patients as a non-invasice approach to exclude coronary disease (Fig. 5.5) (📖 p.46)

Contrast in the myocardium may also be of clinical relevance (Fig. 5.6). Hypo-enhancement is used as a surrogate marker for infarction, especially in the presence of a thinned and akinetic segment of LV. Clinical studies are required to determine if these segments will improve with revascularization or not. Hypo-enhancement in the presence of a normal of hypokinetic segment may represent hibernating myocardium, but further studies are needed. Furthermore, there is interest in imaging the ventricle 3–15 min post contrast injection to look for retained contrast which may represent damaged myocardium, akin to late gadolinium enhancement (LGE).

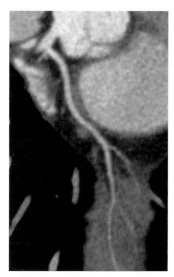

Fig. 5.5 Curved multiplanar reformatted CT coronary angiogram dataset demonstrating left main stem and left circumflex artery.

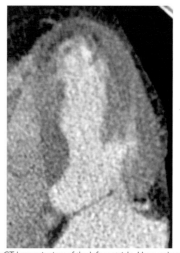

Fig. 5.6 Cardiac CT long-axis view of the left ventricle. Hypo-enhancement is evident in the apex, consistent with an apical infarct.

Cardiac magnetic resonance

Much of the value of CMR is in planning long-term management of a patient who has had a myocardial infarction. This is possible because of the tissue characterization with CMR based around LGE.

- LGE is thought to reflect irreversible (scar) damage to myocardial tissue.
- The spatial resolution of CMR allows detection of LGE in the endo- or epicardial layers.
- Early hypo-enhancement (within 2min of contrast injection) is likely to reflect microvascular obstruction which is also an important indicator of myocardial tissue pathology.

Myocardial infarction (Figs. 5.7 and 5.8)

LGE after myocardial infarction can detect the extent and location of scar. Unsurprisingly, the presence of LGE correlates well with subsequent cardiac events. The spatial resolution is greater than that afforded by SPECT.

Further evaluation of the quality of a myocardial infarction is being undertaken. In particular, CMR is able to differentiate between the necrotic core and a peri-infarct heterogeneous zone which may help in revascularization decisions.

Chest pain—differential diagnoses

CMR is also useful in determining the aetiology of troponin-positive chest pain in the presence of unobstructed epicardial coronaries. The determination of the LGE distribution and pattern helps in the differential diagnosis of myocardial infarction, cardiomyopathy, and myocarditis.

Viability

In CMR, viability is based on the amount of LGE as a proportion of the myocardial wall, i.e. the amount of myocardial tissue that does not take up gadolinium and therefore is functional.

Stress CMR

CMR is increasingly used with stress protocols (p. 142) to look for evidence of perfusion defects and inducible ischaemia.

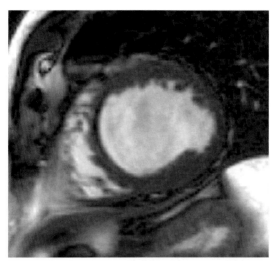

Fig. 5.7 Still image from end-systole during a CMR cine sequence. The image demonstrates a thinned akinetic septum consistent with a myocardial infarction.

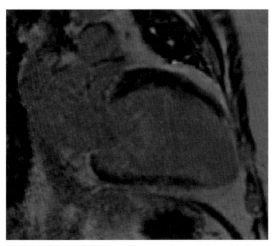

Fig. 5.8 Late gadolinium CMR imaging. The vertical long-axis plane of the left ventricle has highlighted an area of subendocardial enhancement consistent with an apical infarct.

Nuclear cardiology

Chest pain—differential diagnoses

Nuclear cardiology has been tested in the acute setting in patients presenting with symptoms of an acute coronary syndrome but without ECG to prompt PCI and before troponin changes are evident. Nuclear cardiology can then be used to establish whether there is evidence of a perfusion defect that may warrant further invasive strategies. If there is no perfusion defect, the patient may have a speedier discharge from hospital.

Myocardial infarction (Fig. 5.9)

Nuclear cardiology may be useful in the management of myocardial infarction to determine the extent of disease and provide an accurate measure of ejection fraction.

Viability

In nuclear cardiology, viability is based on movement of the wall and the degree of perfusion defect in the territory following stress.

Myocardial perfusion scintigraphy

Myocardial perfusion scintigraphy is a well established technique for assessment of inducible ischaemia (p. 142).

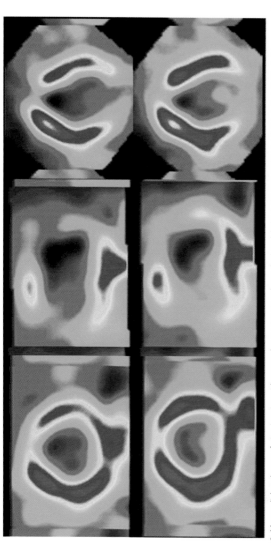

Fig. 5.9 Myocardial nuclear perfusion imaging with rest and stress imaging planes displayed. In both there is evidence of reduced perfusion in the apex and anterior wall consistent with an infarction and an area of non-viable myocardium.

Echocardiography

The advantages of echocardiography are its ease of availability in the acute setting. Echocardiography can also be used in the catheterization laboratory. The image quality is usually sufficient to establish the following.

Myocardial infarction and acute coronary event

- Regional wall motion abnormalities suggestive of an acute reduction in blood supply due to myocardial infarction or ischaemia.
- Ejection fraction as a marker of prognosis following myocardial infarction.
- Additional or alternative diagnoses such as significant valvular disease, aortic dissection, or pericardial effusion.
- Complications of myocardial infarction such as ventricular septal defects, papillary muscle rupture, or pericardial fluid.

Stress echocardiography

Dobutamine stress echocardiography (p. 142) is a major modality used to look for evidence of inducible ischaemia.

Viability

- Viability in echocardiography is often determined by movement at rest. The presence of a thin regional wall (<6mm) is suggestive of a full-thickness myocardial infarct that is unlikely to improve with subsequent revascularization. The segment is usually akinetic.
- Viability can also be determined by *contractile reserve*, i.e. evidence of an improvement in wall motion abnormalities in response to low-dose dobutamine.

Chapter 6

Right ventricle

Right ventricle *154*
Right ventricular structure and function *156*
Echocardiography *158*
Cardiac magnetic resonance *162*
Radionuclide imaging *164*
Cardiac catheterization *166*

Right ventricle

The right ventricle (RV) has gained more interest in recent decades following recognition of its significance in heart failure, pulmonary hypertension, congenital heart disease, and complications of cardiac surgery. However, despite advances in cardiovascular imaging, the RV still causes significant challenges for most of the imaging modalities. Its complex shape and orientation makes it difficult to evaluate using 2D cross-sectional imaging modalities such as 2D echocardiography or radionuclide ventriculography.

Anatomy

The right ventricle lies anteriorly to the left ventricle, and is a complex cavity, more triangular or crescent-shaped than ellipsoid, with thin muscular walls (Fig. 6.1). This distinctive structure allows its anatomical differentiation from the left ventricle, which is especially helpful in diagnosing congenital heart diseases.

Morphological features of the right ventricle

- Presence of a moderator band
- Coarse trabeculation
- Three or more papillary muscles
- Trileaflet configuration of the atrioventricular valve
- Septal leaflet of the tricuspid valve more apical than the anterior leaflet of the mitral valve.

Cardiovascular imaging

The right ventricle presents several challenges for imaging. Echocardiography is the first-line investigation of the right ventricle but for precise measures of size and myocardial structure further imaging with cardiovascular magnetic resonance (CMR) may be required. The reasons for the complexities in imaging the right ventricle are as follows.

- Complex geometry. Currently, there is no universal model for RV geometry, mostly because of its complex shape. This often leads to inaccuracies in volume measurements and a significant variability in measurements obtained with different imaging modalities.
- Complex contraction pattern.
- Heavily trabeculated thin myocardium.
- Several rapidly changing indices of its function.

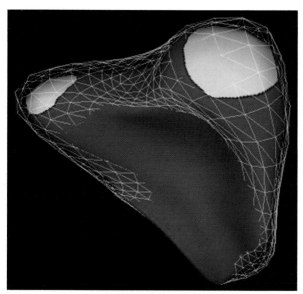

Fig. 6.1 Commercial analysis packages are now able to post-process 3D imaging data files, in particular echocardiographic files, to generate 3D volume reconstructions and functional analysis. In this image, TomTec has been used to generate a 3D volume of the right ventricle.

Right ventricular structure and function

Right ventricular shape and size
The complex shape of the right ventricle creates challenges for geometric modelling in imaging (Fig. 6.2). It also depends significantly on current physiological parameters, and can dynamically adjust to changes in pressure and/or volume. In addition, it is influenced by changes in the left ventricular structure.

Right ventricular function
The right ventricle has approximately one-sixth of the muscle mass and performs against one-tenth of the vascular resistance compared with the left ventricle. Right ventricle systolic function depends on:
- preload
- intravascular volume
- right ventricle compliance
- heart rate
- right atrial function
- pericardial function
- right ventricular contractility
- afterload
- pulmonary resistance
- left ventricular filling.

Right ventricular myocardial blood supply
The right ventricle is supplied mostly by the right coronary artery in the prevalent right-dominant system. A smaller area, mostly in the anteroseptal region, is supplied by the left anterior descending artery.

Ventricular interdependence
As the right ventricle has thinner walls and lower pressure than the left ventricle, it depends strongly on left ventricular function, specifically on interventricular septal changes. In contrast, in the case of significant right ventricular dilatation and a corresponding shift of the interventricular septum to the left, left ventricular function will be influenced by right ventricular function.

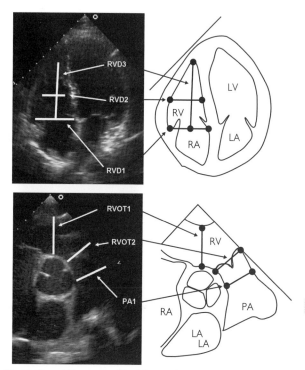

Fig. 6.2 The variable anatomy of the right ventricle means that guidelines have been developed based on multiple measurements of right ventricular size in standardized locations. The figure shows these key measurements of length and width.

Echocardiography

Echocardiography is the most frequently used imaging modality in right ventricular assessment. However, it is often limited by suboptimal views, especially in patients with coexisting pulmonary disease.

Advantages of echocardiography
- Readily available
- Multiple image planes and approaches—subcostal, parasternal, transoesophageal, intracardiac.

Disadvantages of echocardiography
- Difficult ultrasound windows in many patients
- Retrosternal localization of the RV
- Coexisting pulmonary diseases
- Less accurate and less reproducible than CMR and nuclear imaging.

What can echocardiography tell us?

Right ventricular size
Echocardiography provides a rapid assessment of right ventricular size and is often done qualitatively relative to the left ventricle, although quantitative measures are better (Fig. 6.2)

Normally smaller than the left ventricle, the right ventricle can be considered enlarged if the same size or larger than the left.

Right ventricular ejection fraction (RVEF)
Quantitative assessment of the RV systolic function is most frequently based on ejection fraction measurements.

Right ventricular fractional area change (RVFAC)
RVFAC is the ratio of systolic area change to diastolic RV area.
- Planimetry of the RV area is usually performed in the apical four-chamber view (Fig. 6.3)
- The area–length method is more accurate then Simpson's method because it is difficult to acquire appropriate views of the RV for the biplane method in 2D echocardiography.
- Good correlation with ejection fraction.
- Normal range >32%.

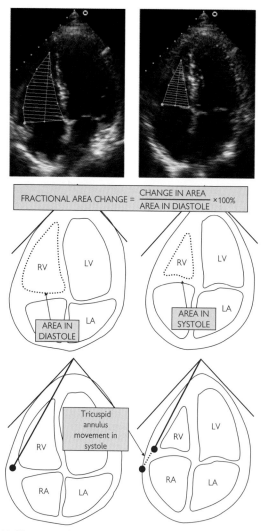

FRACTIONAL AREA CHANGE = $\dfrac{\text{CHANGE IN AREA}}{\text{AREA IN DIASTOLE}} \times 100\%$

Fig. 6.3 2D images can be used to determine function. In this example trans-thoracic echocardiography apical views are used to measure right ventricular ejection fraction based on change in area. An alternative assessment of function can be based on movement of the tricuspid valve annulus (Fig. 6.4). Movement >1cm during systole indicates normal free wall function.

Tricuspid annular plane systolic excursion (TAPSE)

This is one of the most useful quantitative RV systolic parameters. It measures the longitudinal systolic excursion of the lateral tricuspid annulus toward the apex (Fig. 6.4).

- Simple measurement in the apical four-chamber view with M-mode imaging.
- Correlation with overall function of the right ventricle.
- Depends on loading conditions.
- Normal range 15–20 mm.

Strain analysis

Right ventricular strain and strain rate can be assessed similarly to the left ventricle.

- Longitudinal strain can be measured from apical views.
- Radial strain is much more difficult to measure in the right ventricle thin myocardial wall located within thenear field of the ultrasound beam.

Regional wall motion assessment

Segmental right ventricular wall motion abnormalities have been identified in

- Pulmonary embolism
- Acute right ventricular myocardial infarction
- Arrhythmogenic right ventricular dysplasia.

Wall thickness

Gross changes in wall thickness may be evident and can be measured from subcostal views.

Transoesophageal echocardiography (TOE)

Transoesophageal echocardiography plays an important role in the assessment of right ventricular structure and function, especially for:

- perioperative assessment.
  - before surgery for anatomical and functional assessment of the ventricle and valves
  - intraoperative assessment
  - after surgery, especially if there is no access to the precordial region for a transthoracic echocardiogram.
- acutely ill patients in intensive care.

Real-time 3D echocardiography (RT3DE)

RT3DE has a potentially important role because of its ability to acquire 3D datasets of the right ventricle:

- volumetric measurements correlate with CMR
- validation of the method mostly used in highly specialized centres.

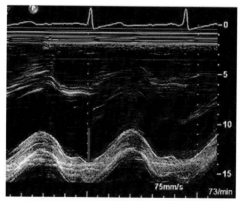

Fig. 6.4 Tricuspid annular plane systolic excursion (TAPSE) provides a measure of RV function. In this example an M-mode trace at the tricuspid lateral annulus has been obtained from an apical four-chamber view and the longitudinal displacement has been measured (indicated by the red line).

Cardiac magnetic resonance

Cardiac magnetic resonance (CMR) is the most accurate method for right ventricular assessment.

Advantages of CMR

- The multiplane/any-plane capability of CMR allows multiple views of the RV walls, as well as RV inflow and outflow, to be obtained in both long and short axes
- It is also possible to study the characteristics of RV myocardium and tissue.

Disadvantages of CMR

- Differentiation between epicardial fat, papillary muscles, and myocardium is more difficult than in LV because of more prominent trabeculation.
- Some applications (e.g. myocardial tagging) are time consuming and limited mostly to clinical research.

What can CMR tell us?

- CMR can image RV morphology and function with high resolution (Figs 6.5 and 6.6).
- Acquisition of the whole RV allows the most accurate volume measurements using standard Simpson's rule.
- Because of the accuracy of volume measurements, ejection fraction measurements are highly reproducible.
- An additional advantage is flow quantification which can be done at the same time as anatomical reconstruction.
- RV mass can be quantified accurately.
- CMR is especially useful for diagnosis of arrhythmogenic RV cardiomyopathy (ARVC):
  - regional wall motion abnormalities
  - adipose tissue replacement.

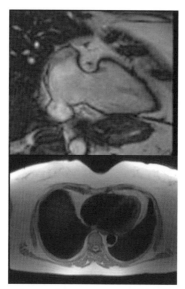

Fig. 6.5 Cardiovascular magnetic resonance images of the right ventricle: right ventricular vertical long-axis view through a normal right ventricle that can be used to assess right ventricular inflow (top); transverse plane through the right ventricle often used to study right ventricular free wall motion and look for evidence of fatty infiltration in ARVC (bottom).

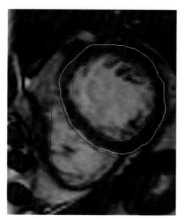

Fig. 6.6 Cardiovascular magnetic resonance can be used to provide accurate measures of right ventricular size through the cardiac cycle. One approach is to use an analysis package to trace the right heart boundaries in multiple short-axis slices from base to apex. Volumes can then be automatically quantified.

Radionuclide imaging

Radionuclide imaging provides adequate and reproducible information about the right ventricular ejection fraction.

Advantages of radionuclide imaging

- It yields the right ventricular ejection fraction on the basis of radioactivity counts and therefore is independent of geometry.
- It is a very well validated imaging technique.

Disadvantages of radionuclide imaging

- A major limitation is the low spatial resolution.
- Low count density with some variables (first-pass technique).
- Difficulties in differentiating counts from planar equilibrium radionuclide ventriculography because of an overlap between cardiac chambers in the standard projections.
- The spatial resolution of SPECT is too low to provide significant information about the right ventricular function. However, sometimes it shows a transient increase in count density within the right ventricle on stress SPECT. This can be seen in global hypoperfusion of the left ventricle.

What can nuclear cardiology tell us?

- Right ventricular ejection fraction.

Cardiac catheterization

As non-invasive techniques like CMR give an accurate estimate of the right ventricular structure, invasive right ventriculography is not commonly performed.

What can catheterization tell us?

- Right heart catherization remains the gold standard for right ventricular haemodynamics:
  - invasive methods provide direct haemodynamic data including assessment of pulmonary vascular resistance.
- Catheterization can provide estimates of the right ventricular volumes. However, there are difficulties related to the lack of accurate modelling of the complex shape of the right ventricle. As a result, catheterization is not used routinely in clinical practice to measure RV volumes.
- Catheterization is occasionally used in the assessment of:
  - tricuspid regurgitation
  - right-to-left shunts
  - right ventricular cardiomyopathies
  - abnormalities of the right ventricular outflow tract.

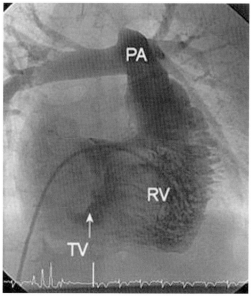

Fig. 6.7 Right ventriculography is not often performed. The figure shows a right ventriculogram from an AP position. The catheter tip is sited in the right ventricle and the pulmonary artery and tricuspid valves are well demonstrated.

Chapter 7

Valves

Valves *170*
Valve structure *172*
Valve function *176*
Valve masses *180*
Severity assessment *184*
Prosthetic valve function *186*
Mitral stenosis *188*
Mitral regurgitation *192*
Aortic stenosis *194*
Aortic regurgitation *198*
Tricuspid valve *200*
Pulmonary valve *202*
Prosthetic valves *204*

Valves

Managing diseases of the four cardiac valves is a major, and growing, feature of cardiology practice. The symptoms of valvular heart disease are well recognized and have been documented for centuries. The stethoscope could be considered as the original 'imaging' device providing critical information on valve disease. To a large extent, the stethoscope has been replaced by current cardiovascular imaging modalities which can now very simply provide elegant detail of the characteristics of valve disease. Therefore imaging of the four cardiac valves must be a key aspect of any cardiovascular imaging modality. Accurate analysis of each valve depends on reliable assessment of:

- valve structure—normal morphology?
- valve motion—leaflet movement normal?
- valve function—stenosis or regurgitation?
- masses—vegetations or thrombus?
- severity assessment—degree of valve lesion?
- additional factors—evidence of cardiac compensation?

Optimal imaging of valves requires high temporal resolution to define valve motion and assess flow accurately, and high spatial resolution to allow identification of calcification and masses such as small vegetations.

Imaging of prosthetic valves follows the same principles, although the presence of artefacts such as metal occluders or sewing rings can limit precise anatomical assessment.

Cardiovascular imaging

The suspicion of valve disease is based upon symptoms and clinical signs, with additional support from initial assessment with ECG and chest X-ray. Imaging of the valves is then required, and typically this is done using transthoracic echocardiography. The major pathologies are narrowing of the valve (stenosis) or leaking of the valve (regurgitation).

In many cases detailed echocardiography is sufficient to confirm the diagnosis and plan management. More complex cases may require further detailed imaging with an alternative modality.

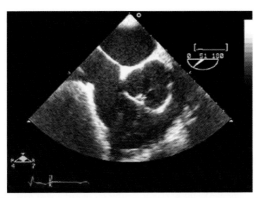

Fig. 7.1 Short-axis view of a normal aortic valve demonstrating three valve leaflets and commisures.

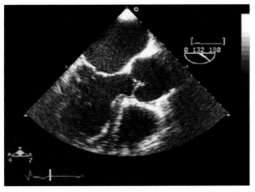

Fig. 7.2 Long-axis view from the same imaging point as in Fig. 7.1. Two of the three leaflets are visible with their attachments to the aortic wall clearly seen. Note that the imaging plane is ~90° from the image in Fig. 7.1.

Valve structure

The assessment of valve structure requires detailed knowledge of normal valve anatomy and an understanding that the 'valve' is far more than just the leaflets. in reality each valve consists of a unique valve 'complex' which may include:

- annulus—the supporting structure of the valve
- leaflets—thin mobile 'cusps' of the valve
- chordae—support the mitral and tricuspid valves
- papillary muscles—secure the chordae to the ventricular mass
- ventricle—crucial to normal function of the atrioventricular valves
- great vessels—sinus of Valsalva is elemental to aortic valve function.

The annulus of the valve is never just a simple circular ring as implied by the name. For example, the 'annulus' of the aortic valve is shaped more like a crown, with three points representing the peaks of the interleaflet triangles formed by the semilunar attachment of each leaflet to the aorta.

The leaflets of the cardiac valves are thin pliable structures which open rapidly to allow unobstructed blood flow and close equally rapidly to minimize regurgitant flow. Leaflet movement also depends on any thickening or abnormality of leaflet tissue. Degenerative calcification of the leaflet body or tips will affect the flexibility of the leaflet.

As the valves consist of a complex of structures rather than the leaflets alone, pathology affecting these areas may affect leaflet movement—for example, prolapse or flail segments of the mitral valve due to disruption of the supporting chordae or papillary muscles.

Assessment of valve structure requires interrogation of all parts of the valve complex and integration of imaging in multiple planes to construct a three dimensional understanding of the size, shape and integration of the components.

- All valves should be imaged in a minimum of two planes, typically a short-axis plane to provide an *en face* view of the valve (Fig. 7.1) and a long-axis plane to examine the valve in line with flow of blood through it (Fig. 7.2).
- The regions above and below the valve itself should also be carefully imaged given their role in valve support and function.

The mitral valve complex is the most challenging to image, given its unique anatomy. In order to visualize all six segments of the valve leaflets additional imaging planes are required, typically with a series of imaging sections rotated around the long axis of the valve.

Imaging valve motion requires high temporal and spatial resolution. This is particularly important for identifying subtle movement abnormalities such as fluttering and timing of valve closure.

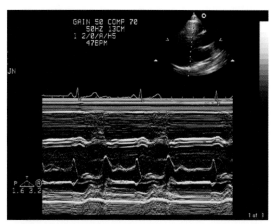

Fig. 7.3 M-mode echocardiography of the mitral valve leaflet tips demonstrating the high detail of leaflet motion.

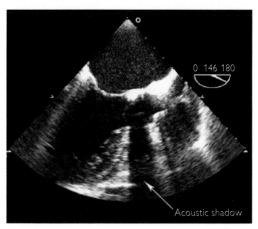

Fig. 7.4 Transoesophogeal echocardiography of calcific aortic stenosis. Note the extensive shadowing behind the calcium obscuring the right coronary cusp.

Echocardiography

M-mode echocardiography affords the highest temporal resolution for fine-detail analysis of valve movement by continuously scanning along only one line. Subtle signs such as fluttering of the anterior mitral valve leaflet due to aortic regurgitation can be detected (Fig. 7.3).

As with valve structure the assessment of valve movement must be done in several imaging planes to ensure that all parts of the valve complex are seen. Marked calcification may cause acoustic shadowing on echocardiography and disrupt imaging of structures beyond the calcium (Fig. 7.4). Alternative imaging planes or the use of transoesophogeal echocardiography may overcome this.

Cardiac magnetic resonance

Cine CMR imaging can provide good visualization of leaflet movement, but the temporal resolution remains lower than that of echocardiography).

Cardiac computed tomography (Fig. 7.5)

Cardiac CT is very useful for demonstrating calcification of valve leaflets (Fig. 7.6), but is not routinely used to assess abnormal leaflet motion.

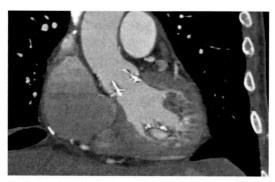

Fig. 7.5 Computed tomography of an aortic valve bioprosthesis (19mm Edwards Perimount). The stent struts are clearly visible but the valve leaflets can hardly be seen.

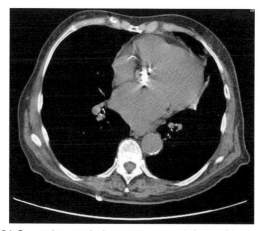

Fig. 7.6 Computed tomography demonstrating severe calcification of the aortic valve.

Valve function

If a valve is structurally abnormal, additional assessment of valve function is mandatory. Is the valve stenotic, regurgitant, or both?

Imaging the high-velocity blood pool as it passes through a valve poses further challenges to the imaging modality. Optimal blood pool imaging will provide data on both flow velocity and direction (Figs. 7.7 and 7.8).

An alternative method of assessing valve function is to measure the orifice of the valve directly. This can be useful in the assessment of stenotic lesions of the aortic and mitral valves. Ensuring that the plani-metered measurement is taken from the leaflet tips and represents the smallest possible orifice is challenging because of movement of the orifice plane during the cardiac cycle.

Many valve lesions will be a combination of stenosis and regurgitation. The effect of the regurgitant jet on forward flow velocity must be understood and integrated into the severity assessment.

If abnormal valve flow is identified, this should be correlated with the valve anatomy. For example, does the regurgitant jet relate to an area of leaflet prolapse?

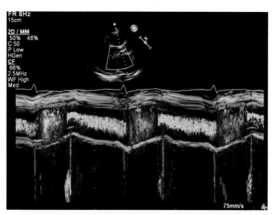

Fig. 7.7 Colour M-mode of aortic regurgitation showing precise definition of onset and duration.

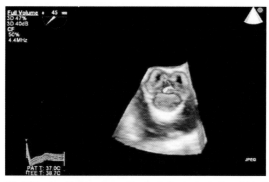

Fig. 7.8 A 3D colour Doppler of an aortic valve in the short-axis plane. A jet of central aortic regurgitation is seen. The apparent holes in two of the valve leaflets are caused by drop-out and are artefacts.

Echocardiography

Doppler echocardiography remains the optimal tool for assessment of valve function and can provide high-resolution information on the speed and direction of blood flow. Continuous-wave, pulsed-wave and colour Doppler are used in combination to provide full details of valve function (Figs. 7.9 and 7.10).

An additional advantage of Doppler echocardiography is the ability to assess flow along a single scan line. This produces a colour M-mode along the line of interrogation and the extremely high temporal resolution (>1000 samples per second) allows precise identification of the timing of onset of flow.

Cardiac magnetic resonance

CMR can assess blood flow using cine phase contrast imaging and provide data on velocity against time for flow through a selected point. A suitable encoding velocity must be pre-chosen to avoid aliasing.

Flow can be visualized either 'through plane' (akin to a short-axis view of the valve) or 'in-plane' (this demonstrates the flow lines along the plane of interest).

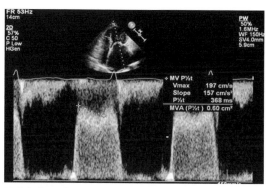

Fig. 7.9 Pulsed-wave Doppler of blood flow through a stenotic mitral valve.
By measuring the rate of velocity decline, and hence the pressure drop across the
valve, the stenotic area can be estimated.

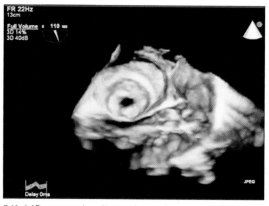

Fig. 7.10 A 3D transoesophageal image of a severely stenotic mitral valve.
A narrow central orifice is visible at the base of a funnel shape formed by the
thickened and abnormal leaflets. This area can be directly measured using
post-processing software.

Valve masses

Identification of abnormal masses attached or adjacent to valves requires similar imaging principles to those for imaging the native valve leaflets. Masses may range from large infective vegetations or tumours to small fine fibrinous strands (Figs. 7.11 and 7.12).

Differential diagnosis of valve masses includes:

- tumour
- infective vegetation
- thrombus
- calcified atherosclerotic mass
- cyst.

Certain features of the mass may aid in identification; for example, vegetations are mobile, irregular, and usually attached to the 'upstream' side of the valve. Tumours such as fibroelastoma may be more uniform and have discrete attachment points.

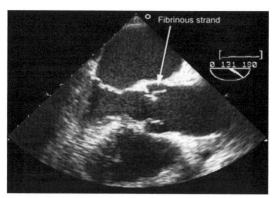

Fig. 7.11 Transoesophageal echo image of an aortic valve with a fibrinous strand arising from the aortic surface of the non-coronary cusp.

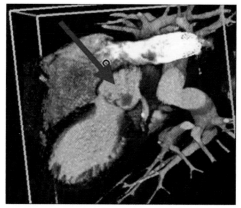

Fig. 7.12 Multislice spiral CT of a papillary fibroelastoma arising from the left coronary cusp. (Reproduced from Bootsveld, A, Puetz J, Grube E (2004). Incidental finding of a papillary fibroelastoma on the aortic valve in 16 slice multi-detector row computed tomography. *Heart* **90**, e35.)

Echocardiography

Both transthoracic and transoesophogeal echocardiography are excellent at imaging valvular masses and are frequently able to clarify the aetiology (Fig. 7.13).

Cardiac magnetic resonance

CMR has the additional advantage of being able to identify if the mass has a blood supply. If the mass enhances to the same degree as myocardium after administration of gadolinium contrast, it is likely to be tumour.

Cardiac CT

Cardiac CT is less suited to soft tissue differentiation, but can provide clear anatomical data and extent of calcification.

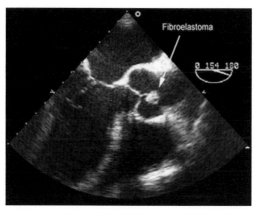

Fig. 7.13 Typical appearance of a papillary fibroelastoma on transoesophogeal echocardiography.

Severity assessment

There are published international guidelines on how to assess the severity of a valve lesion, and many of these relate exclusively to assessment with echocardiography.

The key principle of severity assessment is that no single quantitative measure is used to determine the degree of disease. A number of variables should be assessed and integrated to quantify the valve lesion.

Echocardiography

For stenotic valve lesions the parameters include:
- peak velocity
- valve area—direct planimetry or derived from Doppler data
- peak gradient across the stenosis
- mean gradient across the stenosis.

These quantitative measures, along with a visual assessment of the valve morphology and function, and a search for supportive features (such as left ventricular hypertrophy in aortic stenosis) will then allow accurate assessment of severity.

Multiple valve lesions complicate assessment. For example, concurrent aortic regurgitation will increase forward velocities across a stenotic valve, and mitral stenosis will reduce the forward velocities and may lead to an underestimation of severity.

Another important factor is left ventricular function. The velocity and hence the gradient across the aortic valve depends on the force of the left ventricular ejection. In significant left ventricular dysfunction the measured velocities across a stenotic aortic valve can be very low, even in severe stenosis (Fig. 7.14). This scenario requires more detailed assessment including dobutamine stress echocardiography and transoesophageal echocardiography.

Doppler echocardiography can provide more quantification of valve severity by measuring certain characteristics of colour flow mapping such as the vena contracta—the narrowest portion of regurgitant flow. Assessment of flow velocity upstream of a regurgitant orifice can be used to estimate the area of the regurgitant orifice and regurgitant volume (Fig. 7.15).

Cardiac magnetic resonance

- CMR has the capability to assess flow velocity accurately and to derive gradients as well as planimeter valve area. This is often sufficient to allow accurate classification.
- Given the accuracy of CMR for both left and right ventricular volumes 'indirect' assessment of regurgitant flow can be made by comparing volumes on each side of a diseased valve.

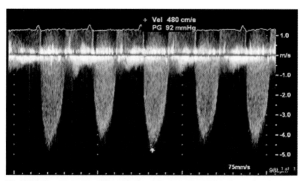

Fig. 7.14 Continuous-wave Doppler through a stenotic aortic valve with a peak velocity close to 5m/s compatible with severe aortic stenosis.

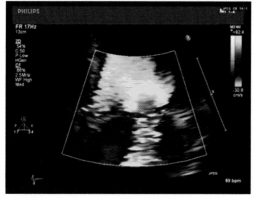

Fig. 7.15 Colour Doppler flow through a regurgitant mitral valve. The settings have been adjusted to allow measurement of the proximal isovelocity surface area from which regurgitant area can be derived.

Prosthetic valve function

Prosthetic valves can be of several types and can pose significant imaging and assessment challenges:

- homograft—human cadaveric valves
- xenograft—biological valves derived from animal tissue
- mechanical—carbon or metal components
- autograft—use of a valve from the patient him/herself (pulmonary valve moved to the aortic valve position).

Imaging of homografts is identical to that of native valves. Most modern bioprosthetic valves (xenografts) have little or no metallic material within the stent supporting the valve leaflets and therefore are usually straightforward to visualize and assess.

Mechanical valves pose a challenge—the large volume of 'reflective' material limits visualization with echocardiography because of the large acoustic shadow beyond the valve. The left atrium can be completely obscured by the acoustic shadow of a mechanical mitral valve during transthoracic echocardiography (Fig. 7.16). This can be overcome by using transoesophageal echocardiography where the left atrium is between the probe and the mechanical mitral valve, and the acoustic shadow now affects the view of the left ventricle (Fig. 7.17).

Prosthetic valves do not produce identical haemodynamics to native valves; furthermore, there is significant variation in effective orifice area, acceptable peak velocities, regurgitant 'washing' jets, and occluder movement patterns between valve design and size. Correct interpretation of the measured data must be referenced to published normal values before any valve dysfunction can be identified.

All modern mechanical prosthetic valves can be safely imaged with CMR (1.5 tesla) although some artefacts will be generated around the valve (Fig. 7.18).

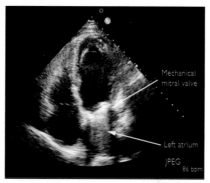

Fig. 7.16 Trans-thoracic echocardiography from the apical position. A mechanical mitral valve casts an acoustic shadow over the whole of the left atrium.

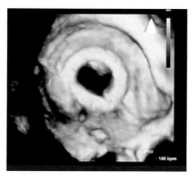

Fig. 7.17 3D Trans-oesophogeal echo of a bioprosthetic mitral valve—the sewing ring is clearly seen and the open valve leaflets are visible.

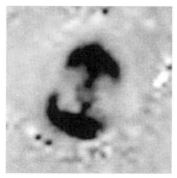

Fig. 7.18 CMR of flow through an open bi-leaflet mechanical prosthesis.

Mitral stenosis

Mitral stenosis is now a rare disease in Western societies, whereas mitral regurgitation is common.

Mitral stenosis is almost exclusively related to prior rheumatic fever caused by group A haemolytic streptococcus infection. It can present as progressive dyspnoea and fatigue or as fulminant heart failure due to sudden decompensation secondary to infection, atrial arrhythmia, or pregnancy.

The murmur of mitral stenosis may be difficult to detect, particularly in sick patients with a low cardiac output. If it is suspected, immediate transthoracic echocardiography is required to confirm and assess severity. Features of mitral stenosis include:

- thickened restricted leaflets
- bowing of anterior mitral leaflet with 'hockey stick' appearance (Fig. 7.19)
- dilated left atrium
- preserved left ventricular function
- pulmonary hypertension
- mitral regurgitation—variable degree.

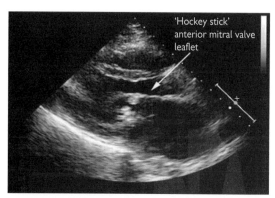

Fig. 7.19 Transthoracic echocardiography demonstrating a markedly thickened and abnormal mitral valve. Note the straight anterior mitral valve leaflet with bowed tip, giving the typical 'hockey stick' appearance.

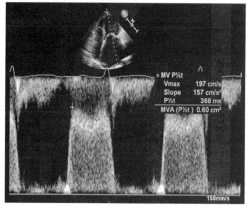

Fig. 7.20 Doppler data for the patient in Fig. 7.19. The rate of decay of the pressure gradient between the left atrium and the left ventricle confirms severe stenosis. The valve area is estimated 0.6cm².

Assessment of severity

The severity of stenosis is related to the estimated area of the valve which can be derived from Doppler data (Fig. 7.20) or by direct visual planimetry. Severe stenosis is defined by a valve area <1cm^2 and a mean pressure gradient across the valve >15mmHg. Significant pulmonary hypertension is expected.

Rheumatic fever can also affect the aortic valve and, rarely, right-sided valves, so a full assessment to exclude any other significant lesions is mandatory.

Treatment options

The preferred treatment option for symptomatic severe mitral stenosis is dilation of the valve with a specialized balloon performed via the venous system and a trans-septal puncture—percutaneous mitral commissurotomy (PMC).

Patients with severe mitral stenosis being considered for PMC require transoesophogeal echocardiography to assess the leaflet morphology, calcification, and degree of regurgitation before proceeding (Figs. 7.21 and 7.22). Surgical valve replacement is required in patients with unfavourable valve anatomy.

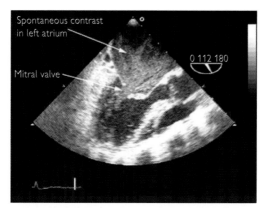

Fig. 7.21 Transoesophogeal echocardiography of severe mitral stenosis. There is also severe spontaneous echo contrast in the left atrium due to near stasis of blood flow.

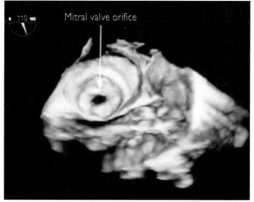

Fig. 7.22 3D transoesophogeal echocardiography viewing the left atrial aspect of the mitral valve with the central elliptical orifice clearly seen.

Mitral regurgitation

Mitral regurgitation is a complex valve lesion as it has a wide variety of aetiologies and mechanisms. Disruption to the function of any part of the mitral valve complex can lead to regurgitation. Commonly encountered scenarios are leaflet prolapse and functional mitral regurgitation as a consequence of ventricular dilation.

Echocardiography

Acute severe mitral regurgitation due to rupture of a papillary muscle complicates a small number of myocardial infarctions but is a medical emergency requiring prompt diagnosis and immediate surgical intervention. Bedside transthoracic echocardiography is the modality of choice in this scenario. Perioperative transoesophageal echocardiography is also a useful aid to surgical planning and assessment of the post-surgical function of the ventricle and valve.

Chronic mitral regurgitation is usually straightforward to identify clinically and is confirmed with transthoracic echocardiography. A standard dataset augmented with quantitative assessment of the regurgitant jet can provide information on:
- leaflet morphology (Figs. 7.23 and 7.24)
- annulus size
- papillary muscle status (Fig. 7.25)
- left ventricular size and function
- left atrial size
- pulmonary hypertension
- effective orifice area and regurgitant volume.

Symptomatic severe mitral regurgitation usually requires surgical intervention, although this depends on the aetiology and function of the left ventricle. Optimum surgical management is repair of the mitral valve where possible, usually involving leaflet reduction and intervention on the chordae, frequently supplemented by annuloplasty with a ring.

All patients referred for consideration of mitral valve repair should undergo transoesophageal echocardiography assessment. This will confirm the aetiology and mechanism of regurgitation along with assessment of the suitability of the valve for repair prior to discussion with the surgical team (Fig. 7.25).

Cardiac magnetic resonance

In cases where the prime mechanism for mitral regurgitation is dilation of the ventricle, CMR is very useful. As well as providing accurate left ventricular volumes and function, the use of gadolinium and delayed imaging can detect myocardial scarring and suggest whether ischaemic cardiomyopathy is the underlying cause. The extent of scar tissue in relation to myocardial thickness can also provide an indication of the likely recovery of myocardial function post revascularization.

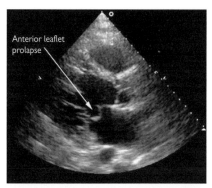

Fig. 7.23 Transthoracic parasternal image of severe prolapse of the anterior mitral valve leaflet.

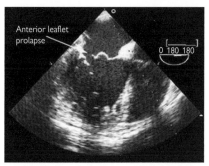

Fig. 7.24 Transoesophogeal view in the patient in Fig. 7.23 confirming severe prolapse of the anterior mitral valve leaflet which is favourable for repair.

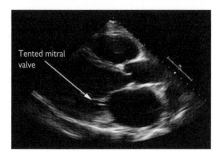

Fig. 7.25 In this example of functional mitral regurgitation dilation of the ventricle has caused traction on the valve leaflets via papillary muscle and chordae displacement. The valve cannot close and an obvious orifice remains even in systole (the aortic valve is open).

Aortic stenosis

Degeneration and calcification of the aortic valve leading to leaflet thickening and stenosis is the most common valve lesion (Fig. 7.26). A congenital abnormality of the valve such as a bicuspid valve (found in ~2% of the population) accelerates this degeneration and patients present at a younger age.

Aortic stenosis typically presents with symptoms of dyspnoea, angina, or syncope, and the clinical signs are easily detected.

Echocardiography

Transthoracic echocardiography is the investigation of choice to assess the morphology of the valve and the severity of the stenosis (Table 7.1), along with documentation of ventricular function and additional valve lesions.

- The severity can be measured by direct planimetry of the valve area but more easily by using quantitative Doppler analysis (Fig. 7.27) to assess the peak pressure drop across the valve and estimating the valve area using the continuity equation. This relies on the principle that the blood flowing through the left ventricular outflow tract (LVOT) will pass through the valve. The LVOT area is measured along with the velocity time integral (VTI) of blood flow at this point. The product of these two is equal to the VTI of the flow through the valve multiplied by the area of the stenotic orifice. The equation can be rearranged to derive the aortic valve area:

    aortic valve area = (LVOT area x LVOT–VTI)/AV–VTI.

- In difficult cases where the valve is hard to image or there are conflicting data on severity, transoesophageal echocardiography is ideal for assessing the valve anatomy in more detail including direct planimetry of the orifice (Fig. 7.28). However, obtaining reliable Doppler data is more difficult because of the challenges in aligning the Doppler beam with flow.
- High velocities along the Doppler beam may appear to come from a stenotic aortic valve orifice, but care must be taken to ensure that there is no subvalvular obstruction (e.g. a membrane or hypertrophic septum) and that the signal is not from an eccentric jet of mitral regurgitation.
- A more complex scenario is aortic stenosis with severe left ventricular impairment. As the flow through the valve depends on the driving force of the ventricle, the peak pressure drop measured may be very low even in severe aortic stenosis. Conversely, the measured pressure drop may be very low due to a poor stroke volume even if the valve is not severely stenosed. Intervention in the valve in this situation would be inappropriate.

Table 7.1 Criteria for assessment of severity of stenosis

Criteria	Mild	Moderate	Severe
Peak instantaneous velocity (m/s)	<3.0	3.0–4.0	>4.0
Peak pressure drop (mmHg)	<35	35–65	>65
Mean pressure drop (mmHg)	<25	25–40	>40
Valve area (cm²)	2.0–1.5	–1.0	<1.0

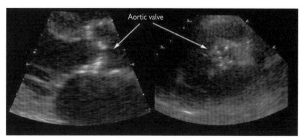

Aortic valve

Fig. 7.26 Parasternal long- and short-axis views of typical aortic stenosis. The leaflets are calcified and restricted with minimal opening in systole.

- If there is doubt over whether the stenosis is truly severe and has caused left ventricular impairment, or is 'pseudo-severe' due to left ventricular impairment itself from another cause, a dobutamine stress echo should be performed.
- Dobutamine will improve the contractility and stroke force of the ventricle if the myocardium is capable of augmenting function. In true severe stenosis this increased stroke volume will lead to an increase in the measured pressure drop across the valve as the orifice is fixed. The estimated valve area will not usually change significantly. In cases of pseudo-severe aortic stenosis valve opening will improve because of increased stroke force and the measured pressure drop will not increase significantly. The estimated valve area will usually increase.
- Stress echocardiography will also provide useful information on the degree of myocardial recovery and aid estimation of the risk of valve replacement surgery and the likely outcome.

Cardiac magnetic resonance and cardiac CT

Further imaging is rarely needed. CT can provide further details of the location and extent of calcification of the valve, annulus, and aorta which may be useful if trans-catheter aortic valve implantation is being considered.

CMR cannot display calcification but can provide accurate assessment of flow velocities through the stenotic valve along with left ventricular volumes, function, and scarring.

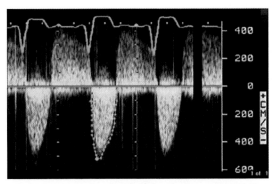

Fig. 7.27 Continuous wave Doppler through the valve shown in Fig. 7.26. The peak velocity is 5.2m/s, implying a peak pressure drop of 109mmHg with a mean of 67mmHg consistent with severe stenosis. There is also aortic regurgitation.

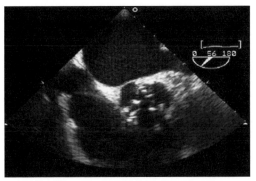

Fig. 7.28 Transoesophogeal echo of a stenotic aortic valve. The thickened and calcified leaflet tips are clearly seen and the restricted orifice is visible.

Aortic regurgitation

The investigation of a regurgitant aortic valve is similar to that of stenosis in that transthoracic and transoesophogeal echocardiography are the first choice.

Echocardiography

A key difference is that aortic regurgitation can present acutely due to abrupt disruption of the valve, usually caused by endocarditis, aortic dissection, or trauma (including iatrogenic). This usually leads to acute severe pulmonary oedema, and is a medical emergency requiring immediate imaging, diagnosis, and management. This is only practical with transthoracic echocardiography (Figs. 7.29 and 7.30).

If aortic dissection is suspected and cannot be identified on transthoracic imaging, CT of the aorta is usually definitive but can delay surgical therapy and expose a potentially unstable patient to limited acute care during the scan. Many advocate transoesophageal echocardiography in the operating theatre under anaesthetic control with provision for immediate surgery if the diagnosis is confirmed.

Chronic aortic regurgitation is well tolerated. Patients are usually monitored using transthoracic echocardiography with careful measurement of left ventricular dimensions and function, as these are key in determining the timing of intervention. It is possible to repair aortic valves and hence patients referred for surgery should undergo detailed examination with transoesophogeal echocardiography.

Cardiac magnetic resonance

Accurate ventricular dimensions and function can be obtained using CMR although all current guidelines refer to measurements obtained from echocardiography.

Nuclear cardiology

Radionuclide ventriculography can also accurately quantify ventricular volumes and function and has been used to monitor patients, including exercise scans to assess for dilation and impairment of ventricular function with effort. This is less commonly used, as accurate echocardiography with echo contrast agents and CMR have become more widely available.

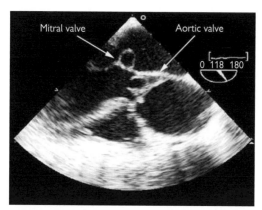

Fig. 7.29 Transoesophogeal echo image of endocarditis affecting both the aortic and mitral valves. There is a large abscess on the aortic valve which has perforated, causing severe aortic regurgitation. The aorta is also dilated.

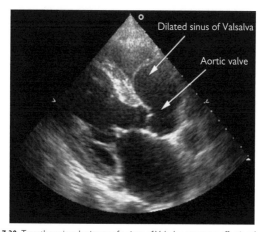

Fig. 7.30 Transthoracic echo image of a sinus of Valsalva aneurysm affecting the right coronary sinus. The dilated sinus has pulled the aortic valve leaflets apart. There is a clear orifice even in diastole (the mitral valve is open), causing significant aortic regurgitation.

Tricuspid valve

Isolated tricuspid valve disease is very rare. A more common problem is tricuspid regurgitation as a consequence of right ventricular dilation and/or dysfunction. This is due to either left-sided valve disease causing pulmonary hypertension and secondary right ventricular dysfunction or intrinsic pulmonary vascular disease.

Therefore one of the most important aspects of assessing tricuspid valve disease is careful assessment of the left-sided valves and estimated pulmonary pressure to identify whether the lesion is primary or secondary. Intervention in a tricuspid valve without relieving the underlying cause will be futile.

Echocardiography

The tricuspid valve is best imaged with echocardiography, with both transthoracic and transoesophogeal echo providing good views of all three leaflets and supporting apparatus (Figs. 7.31 and 7.32).

A degree of tricuspid regurgitation is found in the majority of people and is not pathological unless it is more than mild. A useful feature of this is that the velocity of the tricuspid regurgitation jet into the right atrium is related directly to the peak pressure generated by the right ventricle. If there is no restriction on right ventricular outflow (e.g. no pulmonary stenosis), the peak right ventricular pressure corresponds to the peak pulmonary systolic pressure. As the regurgitant jet flows into the right atrium against right atrial pressure the estimate of peak pulmonary systolic pressure is derived from the peak tricuspid regurgitation velocity plus the right atrial pressure.

Tricuspid stenosis is almost always rheumatic in origin and accompanied by mitral stenosis.

Cardiac magnetic resonance

Detailed assessment of right ventricular volumes and ejection fraction is challenging with echocardiography even if 3D imaging is used. CMR provides more accurate and reproducible measurements of right ventricular function and can also provide data on tissue characterization, such as infarction, myocarditis, or fatty infiltration.

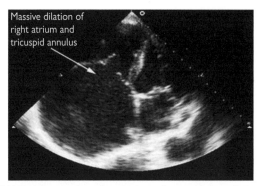

Fig. 7.31 Transthoracic echocardiographic image of severe right heart dilation with a massive right atrium and stretched tricuspid annulus.

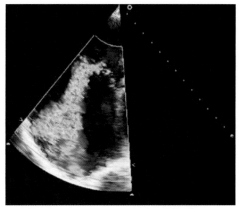

Fig. 7.32 Colour flow mapping of severe tricuspid regurgitation.

Pulmonary valve

Echocardiography

Owing to its anterior location and proximity to lung tissue, the pulmonary valve is the hardest to image with echocardiography. Trans-thoracic imaging can usually provide an adequate view of the long axis of the valve and identify any stenosis or regurgitation (Fig. 7.33). If such a view cannot be obtained from the usual parasternal position, a similar view can be found from a modified subcostal position. It is rare to be able to image the pulmonary valve in the short axis (Fig. 7.34).

Transoesophogeal imaging also affords limited views of the pulmonary valve, but a reasonable long-axis view can be obtained from the oesophogeal or high transgastric position in most patients.

Quantification of the degree of pulmonary regurgitation can be difficult, as can accurate assessment of right ventricular anatomy and function.

Cardiac magnetic resonance

The right ventricular outflow tract or infundibulum is a complex dynamic structure and is best imaged with CMR where the freedom of imaging planes allows accurate views to be obtained in both the long and short axis.

When pulmonary valve disease is suspected, right ventricular size, function and volumes, along with the main and branch pulmonary arteries, require detailed assessment. This can be very challenging with echocardiography and again CMR is more accurate.

Complex surgical and, more recently, percutaneous interventions to the pulmonary valve, infundibulum, and pulmonary arteries are being performed for a variety of pathologies, and these patients require long-term serial imaging to assess the function of any prosthetic device. The dynamic and mobile pulmonary outflow tract places increased stress on valved stents and may lead to fracture. Optimal imaging is likely to be with a combination of echocardiography, CMR and cine fluoroscopy to check for stent integrity.

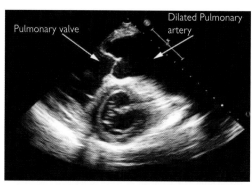

Fig. 7.33 Long-axis view of the pulmonary valve from the parasternal position. This patient had massively dilated pulmonary vessels, making the pulmonary valve much easier to image.

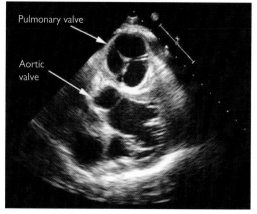

Fig. 7.34 The pulmonary valve shown in Fig. 7.33 could also be imaged in the short axis, clearly demonstrating the three valve leaflets.

Prosthetic valves

Bioprostheses

Imaging of bioprosthetic valves follows the same principle as for native valves. However, older-style valves may have prominent metallic struts forming part of the valve structure which can impair visualization with echocardiography.

Given the variety of style and size of bioprosthetic valves, accurate description of valve function depends on comparing the derived Doppler values with published values. For example, a peak velocity of 3.5m/s would suggest significant stenosis of a native valve, but is normal for a 19mm stented porcine valve.

Ageing bioprosthetic valves demonstrate thickening and reduced leaflet motion leading to stenosis (Fig. 7.35). Regurgitation can occur due to a leaflet tearing from its suspension and becoming flail.

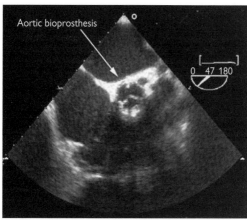

Fig. 7.35 Transoesophogeal image of an aortic bioprosthesis. The three leaflets are clearly visible. Note the subtle thickening of the aortic annulus produced by the sewing ring.

Mechanical prostheses

Imaging of mechanical valves is considerably more challenging because of the artefacts produced by the metal elements (Figs. 7.36 and 7.37). Echocardiography can be very difficult, and a combination of transthoracic and transoesophageal techniques is often required.

If acute valve thrombosis or dysfunction is suspected, echocardiography can identify high gradients across the valve but again these require comparison with manufacturer's normal values.

Cine fluoroscopy is a simple and rapid way of assessing movement of the occluders and can readily identify a 'stuck' leaflet (Fig. 7.38). Thrombus will not be visible at fluoroscopy, but differentiating thrombus from chronic fibrous pannus formation can be very difficult even with a transoesophogeal echo.

CMR can be safely performed in patients with all modern mechanical valves. Artefacts generated from the valve will be seen and can disrupt imaging of local structures.

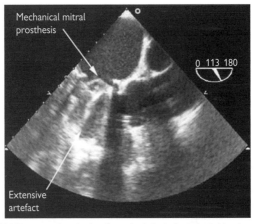

Fig. 7.36 Transoesophageal echo of a mechanical mitral prosthesis. Note how the artefact generated completely obscures the left ventricular cavity and aortic valve.

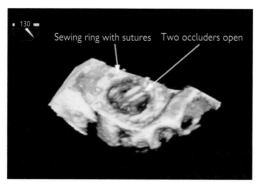

Fig. 7.37 3D transoesophogeal echo of a mechanical mitral prosthesis, clearly demonstrating the sewing ring, sutures and mechanical occluders in the open position.

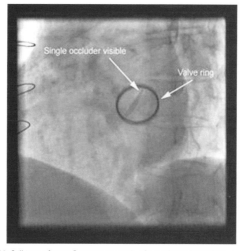

Fig. 7.38 Still image from a fluoroscopic study of a mechanical mitral valve. Only one occluder element is visible in the open position. The other is stuck closed.

Pericardium

Pericardium *210*
Chest X-ray *212*
Echocardiography *214*
Cardiac CT *216*
Cardiac magnetic resonance *218*
Coronary angiography *220*
Nuclear cardiology *220*
Acute pericarditis *222*
Constrictive pericarditis *224*
Pericardial effusion and tamponade *228*
Pericardial tumours *234*
Congenital pericardial disorders *236*
Pericardiocentesis *240*
Pericardiotomy *240*

Pericardium

Introduction
The pericardium stabilizes the heart within the thorax and maintains cardiac efficiency. Pericardial disease is associated with a large range of symptoms from mild discomfort to haemodynamic collapse. Pericardial disease often presents a diagnostic conundrum, and its diagnosis is a good example of multimodality cardiovascular imaging. Echocardiography provides acute assessment of the pericardium, in particular the amount and impact of pericardial fluid. Cardiac CT and MR provide detailed investigation of the pericardial tissue and a wider field of view to look for related disease.

Anatomy
The pericardium consists of a *fibrous pericardium* which superiorly blends into the aorta and pulmonary arteries and inferiorly attaches to the diaphragm, sternum, and vertebrae. Within this is the *serous pericardium*, consisting of two membranes that move over each other lubricated by a small amount of pericardial fluid (10–50mL). There are two holes within the pericardium: one to accommodate the aorta and pulmonary artery, and the other to accommodate the pulmonary veins and vena cavae. Two pockets (or sinuses) are created by these holes: the *transverse sinus* between the aorta and the pulmonary artery, and the *oblique sinus* between the pulmonary veins.

Pathology
Abnormalities of the pericardium have significant haemodynamic consequences because they restrict normal cardiac function.
- The serous membranes provide a potential space for fluid accumulation (*pericardial effusion*) (Fig. 8.1), and increases in intrapericardial pressure related to this fluid can restrict cardiac function (*cardiac tamponade*).
- Changes in pericardial compliance due to fibrosis, such as that associated with chronic inflammation after infection or surgery, can also restrict cardiac function (*constrictive pericarditis*).
- Masses can be found within the pericardium—benign such as pericardial cysts and malignant such as pericardial mesothelioma. These can alter pericardial compliance as well as causing pericardial effusions or direct compression of the cardiac chambers.
- Congenital abnormalities of the pericardium include partial or complete agenesis of the pericardium which may have no functional significance or, if chambers are herniated, may lead to haemodynamic impairment.

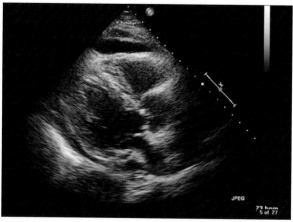

Fig. 8.1 Transthoracic echocardiography subcostal view of a global pericardial effusion. Fluid is evident anterior to the right ventricle and posterior to the left ventricle.

Chest X-ray

As chest X-ray is the standard first-line investigation in patients with chest pain or shortness of breath, this is the usual initial available modality.

Advantages of the chest X-ray

- Widely available.
- Wide field of view to pick up alternative or related pathology such as chest infection.
- Identification of calcification.

Disadvantages of the chest X-ray

- Only provides outline of cardiovascular structures against the lung to identify change in shape. Therefore its main use is in identification of a pericardial effusion which may be confused with other causes for an increased cardiac silhouette.

What can the chest X-ray tell us?

Pericardial disease

- The pericardium itself is not normally visible, except when it becomes calcified. The presence of calcification provides an immediate likely diagnosis of *constrictive pericarditis*.
- Othe irregularities along its border (caused by masses or enlargement of cardiac chambers such as the left atrium in constrictive physiology) and shift of cardiac position within the chest (related to congenital absence of the pericardium).

Pericardial space

The key information is obtained from change in the shape of the cardiac silhouette related to a pericardial effusion (Fig. 8.2). Specific features are:

- increase in size
- a globular heart.

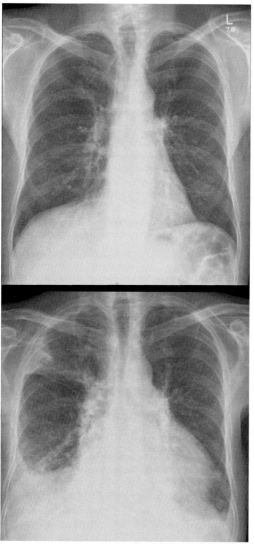

Fig. 8.2 Two chest X-rays in the same patient taken 6 months apart. The top image is normal but the lower image shows that the cardiac shadow has become globular in appearance, consistent with a pericardial effusion.

Echocardiography

Echocardiography is the initial imaging modality of choice for investigation of possible pericardial pathology.

Advantages of echocardiography

- Readily available within the hospital.
- High spatial and temporal resolution to provide information on the quantity and position of fluid within the pericardial space combined with related changes in haemodynamics.
- Can also assess cardiac size, function, and mass.
- Transoesophageal imaging can also assess sinuses.
- Some tissue characterization (e.g. the presence of thrombus or fibrin in effusion or masses associated with the pericardium) can be identified. Useful in the emergency setting to assess acute haemodynamic compromise and assist with pericardial drainage.
- Doppler can assess both myocardial and blood velocities to investigate constrictive and restrictive physiology.

Disadvantages of echocardiography

- Field of view does not allow study of related pathology in the chest.
- Imaging may be limited by body habitus.
- Limited ability to study tissue characteristics of any pericardial masses.
- Not able to accurately measure pericardial size.

What can echocardiography tell us?

Part of the pericardium and pericardial space is seen in all standard echocardiography views. Echocardiography is used to identify masses or calcification and accumulation of fluid within the pericardial space. It can be combined with Doppler assessment of valvular flow during respiration to assess cardiac compromise. At the same time a comprehensive assessment of cardiac and valvular function can be performed.

- The best views are the parasternal long- and short-axis, apical four-chamber, and subcostal views (Fig. 8.3).
- During transoesophageal echocardiography additional views are available, including the four-chamber view (mid-oesophageal 0° view) to assess localized collections around the pulmonary veins and right heart.
- Pericardial surfaces are seen as a thin, slightly brighter line around the heart, but the acoustic properties of the pericardium are similar to surrounding tissue and therefore are difficult to measure accurately. Gross changes in thickness or calcification (which are seen as echo-lucent areas with associated shadowing) may be apparent.
- Pericardial space is seen as a thin black line around the heart, which is usually only a few millimetres thick.

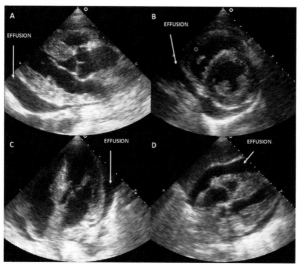

Fig. 8.3 Four standard echocardiography views with the pericardial effusion annotated.

Cardiac CT

Cardiac CT is a key modality for more detailed assessment of pericardial pathology that has been identified by echocardiography. Pericardial disease may also be identified during chest CT imaging for investigation of symptoms such as shortness of breath. As the modality has been available for longer than magnetic resonance imaging, it has traditionally been the modality of choice for detailed assessment of pericardial pathology. Multi-detector CT has enabled motion-free imaging of the pericardium to improve resolution, multiplanar re-formation, and options to assess associated changes in cardiac function.

Advantages of cardiac CT

- Ability to provide soft tissue contrast with tissue characterization based on attenuation.
- Ientification of calcification, including microcalcifications (Fig. 8.4).
- Wide field of view allowing identification of associated chest pathology.

Disadvantages of cardiac CT

- Without gating, motion artefacts can make measurements difficult including complicating differentiation of thickened pericardium from fluid.
- Requirement for ionizing radiation.
- Use of iodinated contrast agents.

What can cardiac CT tell us?

- Pericardial surfaces are seen as a thin grey line of soft tissue density. This is predominantly fibrous pericardium but also incorporates the serous membranes. The presence of pericardial and epicardial fat improves delineation of the pericardium because of the attenuation characteristics of fat. Therefore thickness is best assessed in front of the right ventricle and right atrium where there is an area of ventral mediastinal fat. Thickness is usually 1–2mm, with >4mm considered abnormal (Fig. 8.5). Calcifications suggest constrictive pathology.
- Pericardial fluid has the attenuation characteristics of water and is seen as a thin line between the pericardial surfaces and the heart. Attenuation characteristics may allow differentiation between transudates (attenuation similar to water) and exudates or haemorrhage (higher protein content with greater attenuation). Because the whole heart is seen, loculated or localized effusions can be imaged.
- Multi-detector CT allows visualization of cardiac function to identify chamber collapse or changes in cardiac chamber size.
- The wide field of view allows assessment of related pathology in the lungs and clearer characterization of the extent of masses associated with the pericardium. Therefore cardiac CT is particularly useful for more detailed assessment of pericardial pathology, in particular pericardial thickness, calcification, and size, and the extent and functional effects of pericardial masses.

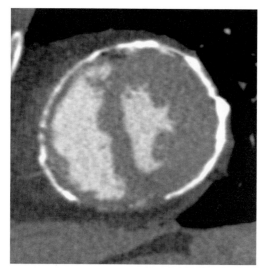

Fig. 8.4 Cardiac CT short axis view of the left ventricle. Pericardial calcification consistent with constrictive pericarditis is easily seen.

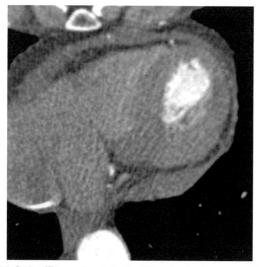

Fig. 8.5 Cardiac CT image of a patient with a thickened pericardium seen as a thick line around the cardiac shape. The thickened pericardium is easy to see because a pericardial effusion is also present (black line dividing the pericardium from the heart).

Cardiac magnetic resonance

Cardiac magnetic resonance (CMR) imaging is increasingly used as the modality of choice for more detailed assessment of pericardial pathology.

Advantages of CMR

- Unrestricted planes of view.
- Differentiation of tissue and fluid characteristics based on T_1 and T_2 characteristics.
- Functional cardiac imaging.
- Assessment of myocardium to investigate cardiomyopathic processes that may complicate differentiation of constrictive and restrictive physiology.
- Wide field of view allowing study of related chest pathology or definition of extent of pericardial masses.
- Avoids ionizing radiation.

Disadvantages of CMR

- Investigations are relatively time consuming.

What can CMR tell us?

- Pericardial surfaces are visible as a thin dark line on most CMR sequences (T_1 and T_2 weightings, steady state free precession (SSFP) imaging) surrounding the heart. It is dark on both T_1- and T_2-weighted sequences because it is fibrous with a low water content. Fat has different characteristics, and therefore pericardial and epicardial fat help delineate the pericardium. The pericardium is best seen adjacent to the right ventricle, whereas it is least visible by the inferolateral wall of the left ventricle because of the presence of the low-intensity lung. Normal thickness is 1–2mm, which probably includes some of the surrounding fibrous tissue as this is greater than pathological measurements.
- Pericardial fluid is visible as a dark rim on T_1 weightings and high intensity on T_2 weightings or SSFP imaging (Figs. 8.6 and 8.7). It is strikingly black on late enhancement images. Loculated effusions, particularly around the aortic–pericardial reflection and at the left ventricular apex, can be seen using the wide field of view. Transudates (normal pericardial fluid) have a low signal on T_1 and a high signal on T_2, whereas exudates have a higher signal on T_1. Inflammatory or protein-rich material can create patchy changes in signal intensity.
- The size and extent of pericardial masses and tissue characteristics can be used to aid diagnosis of pericardial masses.
- Cine images of cardiac function and free-breathing sequences allow identification of haemodynamic changes such as chamber size and collapse associated with pericardial fluid.

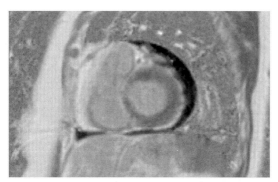

Fig. 8.6 CMR late gadolinium imaging. On these sequences a pericardial effusion appears as a black areas around the heart.

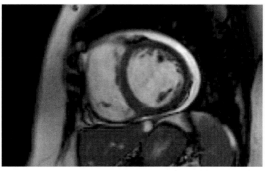

Fig. 8.7 On a standard CMR SSFP cine image a transudate pericardial effusion appears bright white.

Coronary angiography

The cardiac silhouette can be seen during angiography, and therefore changes in size may provide a clue to collection of pericardial fluid. In iatrogenic pericardial effusion following intervention the pericardial space may become evident due to accumulation of contrast around the heart. During pericardiocentesis, contrast injected purposefully into the pericardial space during fluoroscopy can be used to confirm needle position. The pericardium itself is not seen although calcification may be noted.

Nuclear cardiology

The pericardium is not seen on nuclear perfusion imaging. FDG-PET measures metabolic activity and therefore changes in uptake within the pericardium can occur in pericardial tumours or in chronic inflammatory pericarditis. However, it is not used as a clinical tool as it is usually difficult to distinguish uptake from that seen in the myocardium.

Acute pericarditis

Acute pericarditis describes acute inflammation of the serous membranes and is associated with sharp chest pain, which varies with respiration. Pericarditis can be caused by infections (bacterial or viral), myocardial infarction, uraemia, or radiation damage. An acute inflammatory reaction within the pericardium can also occur after cardiac surgery (post-cardiotomy syndrome).

X-ray and echocardiography

Chest X-ray and echocardiography are routinely performed in those in whom acute pericarditis is one of the differential diagnoses.

- Inflammation of the pericardium cannot be seen with X-ray.
- Echocardiography is not diagnostic. Although the pericardium is meant to be 'brighter' this is not a reliable sign.
- These modalities can be useful for investigating the complications of pericarditis such as effusions or associated pathology (changes in cardiac function following myocardial infarction or myocarditis).
- If echocardiography identifies significant pathology underlying the acute pericarditis, more detailed assessment by CMR and cardiac CT can be undertaken.

Cardiac CT and CMR

These modalities are usually not warranted for diagnosis or management of acute pericarditis unless other pathology needs to be investigated. It may be possible to identify acute pericardial thickening associated with acute pericarditis with CMR or cardiac CT. In this situation the normally smooth contour can become irregular, and it has also been reported that the inflamed pericardium enhances following gadolinium contrast (Fig. 8.8).

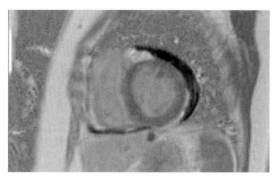

Fig. 8.8 In this CMR late gadolinium image there is some evidence of gadolinium uptake in the pericardium making it white. This finding is consistent with pericardial inflammation as may occur with percarditis.

Constrictive pericarditis

Constrictive pericarditis is uncommon, and often presents with vague signs and symptoms with a long history. It is usually due to chronic inflammation as a result of infection (classically tuberculosis), cardio-thoracic surgery, radiation, or connective tissue disease. Chronic inflammation causes fibrosis, a reduction in pericardial compliance, and, in severe forms, adherence of the pericardium to the myocardium. Acute pericardial inflammation can also cause similar transient findings. The loss of pericardial compliance leads to impaired relaxation of the heart and constrictive physiology. Diagnosis is usually clinical, based on history and signs, with imaging used to confirm the diagnosis and plan surgery if required. A common diagnostic dilemma is differentiation between constrictive pericarditis and a restrictive cardiomyopathy. Clinically, both may have similar symptoms and imaging can powerfully aid diagnosis (Fig. 8.9).

Chest X-ray

Chest X-ray may demonstrate pericardial calcification, diagnostic of chronic pericarditis. More likely it will demonstrate a normal cardiac size in someone with clinical symptoms of shortness of breath. A normal chest X-ray should not exclude the possibility of constrictive pathology.

Echocardiography

Echocardiography is the modality of choice for initial investigation of constrictive pericarditis. Doppler will demonstrate haemodynamic changes and myocardial function. Echocardiography also provides a rapid means of excluding other pathology that may account for breathlessness such as impaired left or right ventricular systolic function or valvular disease.

- The thickened pericardium may be visible, and may appear bright or demonstrate calcifications (dark areas with shadowing distally).
- Systolic function should be normal. If it is not, investigation for other causes of the symptoms should be pursued.
- Septal motion may be abnormal with fluttering of the septum as left and right ventricles fill during diastole, probably due to waves of competitive filling of the two ventricles. This is seen as early diastolic notching on M mode.
- Doppler findings are similar to those associated with tamponade but without evidence of diastolic ventricular collapse. Features of diastolic dysfunction are also evident, for example an exaggerated E/A ratio on mitral inflow and shortened deceleration time. However, tissue Doppler imaging demonstrates normal myocardial motion. Increases in filling pressures may also lead to increases in the size of atria, coronary sinus, inferior vena cava and hepatic veins.

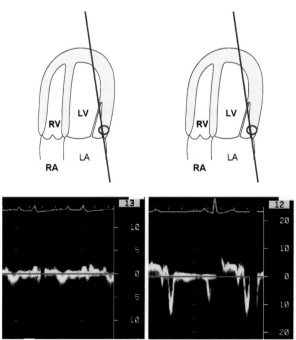

Fig. 8.9 To differentiate constrictive pericarditis from restrictive cardiomyopathy tissue Doppler imaging of the mitral annulus can be used to determine whether there is normal myocardial motion (suggestive of constrictive physiology) (right image) or restricted motion (suggestive of restrictive cardiomyopathy) (left image).

The key imaging features of constrictive pericarditis are as follows.
- *Pericardial thickening and possibly calcification* The pericardium can thicken up to 1cm and is very often focally thickened. Thickening and compression of the right ventricle more common than that of the left. Patterns of thickening have been classified as global, annular, left-sided, right-sided, epicardial, or effusive. Location of thickening is required to aid surgical planning if pericardial removal is considered.
- *Changes in cardiac function and chamber size* Imaging can be used to confirm the presence of constrictive pericarditis, rather than restrictive cardiomyopathy, by demonstrating that there is abnormal diastolic filling without evidence of a cardiomyopathy. Thickening can occur in the absence of constrictive physiology, and findings need to be interpreted based on clinical symptoms. Conversely, if the pericardium is not thickened, constrictive physiology is less likely, but it cannot be excluded as the pericardium may be stiff because of previous pericarditis without significant thickening.

Cardiac CT

The particular strengths of cardiac CT are its ability to identify calcifications, even microcalcifications, in the pericardium and to assess pericardial thickening accurately. Functional cardiac CT may also give some information on changes in cardiac function or alternative pathologies.

- Calcifications are seen as bright white areas within the pericardial layer surrounding the heart. Windowing can be optimized for the calcifications. Calcium within the pericardium in someone with clinical symptoms consistent with constrictive pericarditis makes the diagnosis highly likely.
- Pericardial thickening and its location can be measured.
- Cardiac function assessment during cardiac CT can be used to confirm normal left ventricular systolic function and changes in septal motion indicative of constrictive physiology.

Cardiac magnetic resonance

CMR provides accurate information on pericardial thickness and location of thickening, but not on calcification. Particular strengths of the technique are its ability to generate information on cardiac size and function alongside detailed assessment of the myocardium to exclude cardiomyopathic processes associated with restrictive cardiomyopathy.

- Location and extent of pericardial thickening can be determined.
- Cine imaging can be used to identify the classic early diastolic abnormalities in septal motion with normal left ventricular function. Free-breathing sequences may demonstrate septal flattening on inspiration consistent with the haemodynamic variation measured with Doppler during echocardiography and the disappearance of vena caval collapse on inspiration suggestive of increased right atrial pressure.
- The atria may be dilated along with the IVC and coronary sinus.
- CMR provides an opportunity to determine whether there is evidence of a restrictive cardiomyopathy. This can be based on evidence of left-ventricular hypertrophy with patterns of late enhancement following gadolinium to suggest an infiltrative pathology. These techniques may also identify alternative diagnoses such as ischaemia.

Pericardial effusion and tamponade

Pericardial effusions

Pericardial effusions vary significantly in size and haemodynamic effect, and the two factors are not related. Haemodynamic effects are more closely related to speed of fluid accumulation. Effusions typically occur in response to pericardial inflammation, as part of a malignant process, associated with metabolic changes, or due to abnormalities in drainage such as a chylous effusion. Haemopericardium occurs if there is pathological or iatrogenic cardiac or coronary rupture. Localized effusions occur after cardiac surgery (blood) or infections (loculation).

Cardiac temponade

Cardiac temponade is a clinical diagnosis based on tachycardia (>100bpm), hypotension (<100mmHg systolic), pulsus paradoxus (>10mmHg drop in blood pressure on inspiration) and a raised jugular venous pressure with prominent x descent. Cardiac temponade occurs when an effusion causes sufficient increase in intrapericardial pressure to restrict normal blood flow through the heart (Fig. 8.10).

Echocardiography is the initial modality used in management of pericardial effusions, with cardiac CT and CMR reserved for patients where there is a need to investigate possible underlying diagnoses. Cardiovascular imaging should be used to identify the following.
- The size and location of the effusion. Global effusions are graded as mild, moderate, or large based on depth of fluid.
  - minimal <0.5cm or 50–100mL
  - mild: 0.5–1cm or 100–250mL
  - moderate: 1–2cm or 250–500mL
  - large: >2cm or >500mL
- The likely cause. Intrapericardial structures may point to diagnosis such as fibrin strands (inflammation), haematoma (haemopericardium), irregular/invasive masses (tumour, cyst, or fungal infection).
- Haemodynamic effects. Cardiac temponade leads to right atrial and ventricular collapse, and the appearance of a swinging right atrium and ventricle. The change in flow through the heart can also be demonstrated with Doppler recordings.
- The best approach to removing the effusion (pericardiocentesis).

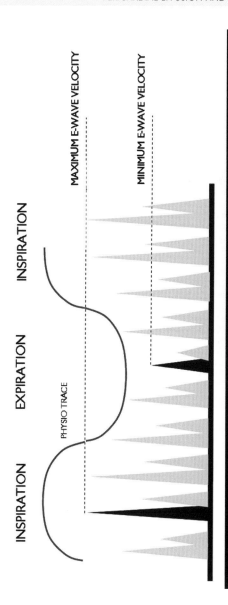

Fig. 8.10 In cardiac tamponade there is an exaggerated variation in flow through the heart with respiration (this is clinically recorded as pulsus paradoxus). This can be demonstrated most easily with echocardiography at the tricuspid or mitral valve using pulsed-wave Doppler with a physiological trace to document respiration.

Chest X-ray

The classical feature of an effusion on chest X-ray is an enlarged globular heart. This should prompt further imaging. Chest X-ray may inform on possible underlying or alternative pathologies such as the chest infections, tuberculosis, or malignancy.

Echocardiography

Echocardiography is the modality of choice for initial assessment of pericardial effusion and, in particular, cardiac tamponade because this is often an acute problem and the high temporal resolution means that image quality is not affected by movement of the heart within the fluid (swinging heart).

- Echocardiography can allow approximation of volume of fluid based on depth.
- It may be difficult to determine nature of pericardial fluid (serous, blood or pus) are all seen as black echolucent areas. Strands (fibrin) can easily seen and haematoma may be evident although it has similar echocardiographic density to myocardium.
- Transoeosphageal echocardiography may be particularly useful for assessment of possible localized effusions in patients with haemodynamic problems after cardiac surgery.
- Echocardiography will identify the characteristic right atrial and ventricular collapse of cardiac tamponade (Fig. 8.11). Furthermore, Doppler provides a means to demonstrate the pulsus paradoxus used clinically to diagnose tamponade. Normally peak flow across the mitral valve varies by <15% and <25% at the tricuspid valve. Greater than this supports tamponade but clinical signs are usually associated with >40% variation at the mitral valve.

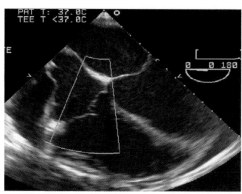

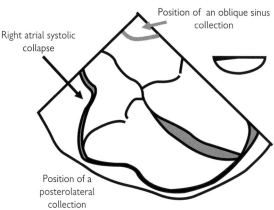

Position of an oblique sinus collection

Right atrial systolic collapse

Position of a posterolateral collection

Fig. 8.11 Transoesophageal echocardiographic four-chamber view demonstrating right atrial collapse associated with the pericardial effusion.

Cardiac CT

- Cardiac CT can be used to assess loculated effusions or localized effusions that are not well visualized on echocardiography.
- CT may be indicated to investigate underlying causes such as malignancy.
- Effusions may be identified on CT. Transudates have the attenuation of water, whereas those with higher protein content, such as haemo-pericardium, purulent exudates, malignancy, or chylous effusions, have high attenuation. The attenuation of haemopericardium varies with age and gradually reduces over time with emergence of mixed areas due to thrombus. Inflammatory effusions may be associated with pericardial contrast uptake.
- Differentiation of a small effusion from pericardial thickening or when the effusion is the same attenuation as pericardium may be difficult.
- Cardiac tamponade should have been identified. However, when present during CT examination it is associated with changes in cardiac chamber appearances, as described for echocardiography.

Cardiac magnetic resonance

- CMR can be used to study associated, additional, or alternative diagnoses.
- CMR will provide information on the nature of pericardial effusions. Transudates have a low signal on T_1 and a high signal on T_2, with complex exudative effusions exhibiting greater signal intensity on T_1. SSFP cine imaging is associated with greater signal intensity in the presence of a greater T_2/T_1 ratio, and therefore transudates tend to have high intensity. Effusions do not take up contrast and appear black on both early and late enhancement imaging.
- If cardiac tamponade is present, the classical right heart signs of ventricular and atrial collapse can be imaged and should prompt referral for treatment (Fig. 8.12).

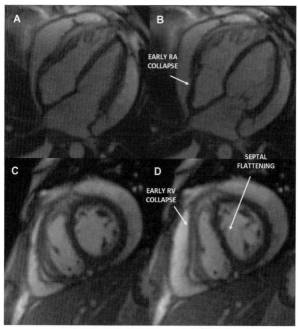

Fig. 8.12 Still images from a real-time CMR free-breathing sequence demonstrating right atrial and right ventricular collapse, as well as septal flattening, during respiration consistent with cardiac tamponade.

Pericardial tumours

Primary pericardial tumours are rare. The most common is mesothelioma, with fibrosarcoma, angiosarcoma, and malignant teratoma being less common. More commonly tumours invade from the mediastinum or lungs and are associated with effusions and possible tamponade. Sarcoma, lipoma, and haemangioma can also occur within the pericardium. Pericardial metastases occur 40–60 times more frequently than primary tumours. However, in 42% of patients with malignancy who had peri-cardial complications (e.g. effusion) there was no direct pericardial involvement by tumour. Cardiovascular imaging is used for the following purposes.

- Definition of the size and extent of pericardial tumours. Although echocardiography is useful for identifying their presence, cardiac CT or CMR is essential for comprehensive assessment.
- Assessment of the haemodynamic effects of tumours.

Chest X-ray

Chest X-ray may demonstrate cardiac enlargement with irregular contours as well as possible associated pericardial effusion and mediastinal enlargement. If the cause is metastatic disease there may be evidence of metastatic deposits, such as bones, or a primary lung tumour may be evident.

Echocardiography.

- Echocardiography may pick up irregular thickening of the pericardium and demonstrate whether the tumour is contained within the pericardium or has invaded the myocardium.
- Differentiation of whether masses lie within or outside the pericardium and the tissue characteristics of tumours is difficult.
- Transthoracic echocardiography may miss tumours lying posterior to the heart and does not allow identification of other metastatic deposits or the presence of primaries elsewhere.
- A strength of echocardiography is its ability to assess the haemodynamic effects of tumours and if there has been invasion into the myocardium. Intracardiac echocardiography can aid myocardial biopsy.

Cardiac CT

- Cardiac CT provides a more definitive assessment of pericardial tumours as it allows description of size, location, extra-pericardial extension, and irregularities of the thickened pericardium.
- Imaging can be combined with assessment of the chest and mediastinum to identify other tumour deposits and lymph node involvement.
- Attenuation characteristics of the masses may also provide some information on likely diagnosis; for instance, lipoma has low attenuation on CT, whereas lymphoma, sarcoma, and liposarcoma typically appear as large heterogenous masses with serosanguinous effusions.

Cardiac magnetic resonance

- CMR can easily demonstrate pericardial tumours and characterize their haemodynamic significance. The pericardium will appear irregularly thickened, and loss of the pericardial line confirms the pericardial involvement or origin.
- The ability of CMR to distinguish tissue characteristics can be particularly useful. Malignant areas usually enhance following contrast because of their vascularity, whereas normal pericardium or cysts will not. Most neoplasms have a low signal intensity on T_1 weightings and high signal on T_2, apart from metastatic melanoma which has high signal intensity on T_1 weightings. Lipomas have a high signal intensity on T_1 weightings, and the presence of patchy calcium or fat within a pericardial mass is suggestive of teratoma. Fibromas have a low signal intensity on T_2 and do not enhance.

Congenital pericardial disorders

Cysts

Pericardial cysts are the most common pericardial mass. They are usually benign and asymptomatic. They can cause chest discomfort, shortness of breath, cough, or fever. They are usually in the cardiophrenic angle but may be elsewhere in the mediastinum. 90% are in contact with the diaphragm, 65% in the right cardiophrenic angle, 25% on the left, and 10% are higher. Confusion may arise between a pericardial cyst and a cyst within the lungs or thymus. As with pericardial masses, echocardiography is usually used to identify the presence of cysts, with cardiac CT or CMR used to provide definitive assessment.

Chest X-ray

Chest X-ray may demonstrate an irregular cardiac border. However, this depends on the position of the cyst within the pericardium and there may be little to see on chest X-ray.

Echocardiography

Pericardial cysts are seen as echolucent rounded masses lying attached or within the pericardium (Fig. 8.13). Echocardiography can be used to assess the haemodynamic effects of the mass, but further imaging is warranted to define the extent of the cyst.

Cardiac CT

Cardiac CT can very effectively highlight pericardial cysts as rounded smooth thin-walled masses lying close to the cardiac border (Fig. 8.14). They usually have no internal septa, and the central attenuation characteristics differ from the wall consistent with the cyst's being fluid-filled. The attenuation is likely to be the same as that of water and does not enhance following contrast.

Cardiac magnetic resonance

CMR will demonstrate cysts associated with the cardiac border and can be used to determine whether the cyst lies within or outside the pericardium. The cyst should classically contain fluid and have low or intermediate intensity on T_1-weighted images with high intensity on T_2 or SSFP images. If the cyst contains proteinaceous material, it will tend towards higher intensity on sequences with more weighting towards T_1.

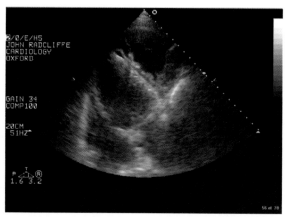

Fig. 8.13 Transthoracic echocardiography apical view of patient with pericardial cyst showing the potential localization of pericardial pathology.

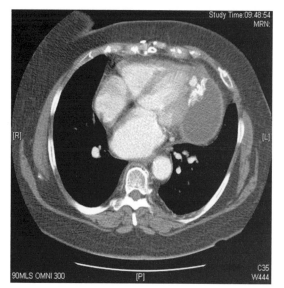

Fig. 8.14 Cardiac CT transverse plane through the heart. A pericardial cyst is present adjacent to the apical segment of the lateral wall of the left ventricle. Calcification is also evident within the pericardium at the site of the cyst.

Congenital absence

This condition is rare and is thought to relate to problems with blood supply to the pleuro-pericardial membrane during development. The patient may be asymptomatic or, particularly if there is only partial absence, there may be acute problems associated with herniation. The key findings on imaging are:

- physical absence of the pericardium and an abnormal shape or position of the heart
- coexisting congenital abnormalities.

Therefore cardiac CT and CMR are important to define the extent of disease.

Chest X-ray

Absence of the pericardium is associated with changes in the cardiac silhouette, in particular leftward displacement of the heart and aorta, with a flattened silhouette and prominent pulmonary artery. Typically there is a radiolucent band between the left hemi-diaphragm and the base of the heart.

Echocardiography

Echocardiography provides rapid initial assessment, with the most obvious finding being herniation of part of the heart. This often involves the left or right atrial appendage or parts of the ventricle. As on radiography, the heart may be abnormally positioned with right atrial or ventricular dilatation and paradoxical septal motion. Further more detailed imaging is indicated.

Cardiac CT

Absence of the pericardium is suspected when it is not possible to identify the fibrous pericardial layer along the left cardiac border, with a change in axis of the main pulmonary artery and direct contact between the lung and the cardiac surfaces. A classic feature is interposition of lung tissue between the aorta and pulmonary artery.

Cardiac magnetic resonance

The findings are similar to those seen on cardiac CT with lung between aorta and pulmonary artery as well as difficulty in identifying the pericardium. Functional changes or herniation of the heart are also easy to identify.

Pericardiocentesis

Pericardiocentesis is used to drain pericardial effusions for diagnostic purposes or to treat cardiac tamponade. Cardiovascular imaging is used to guide needle insertion and monitor fluid removal.

Chest X-ray and angiography

Fluoroscopy can aid pericardial drainage because the needle is clearly seen on screening. The needle can be followed according to the landmarks of the ribs and spine to a position where the pericardial space should be present. Injection of a small amount of iodinated contrast is sometimes used to demonstrate that the needle is in the pericardial space.

Echocardiography

- Echocardiography is the modality of choice for imaging guided pericardiocentesis.
- Pericardiocentesis is usually performed from the subcostal or apical positions and echocardiography allows evaluation of location and depth of fluid in each location.
- The angle of the echo probe used to achieve images can be used as a guide to the angle to be used for the needle.
- Imaging during the procedure can sometimes be used to identify the needle advancing into pericardial space and to confirm the position by injection of a small amount of agitated saline contrast down the needle (Fig. 8.15).

Pericardiotomy

Imaging is used for preoperative evaluation to establish what the surgeon will find and where it is best to remove the pericardium. Cardiac CT or CMR are the modalities of choice to achieve these aims because of their wide field of view, unlimited scan planes, 3D reconstructions, and accurate in measurement of pericardial thickness. Transoesophageal echocardiography can be used to monitor cardiac function during the procedure and to ensure resolution of haemodynamic effects before chest closure.

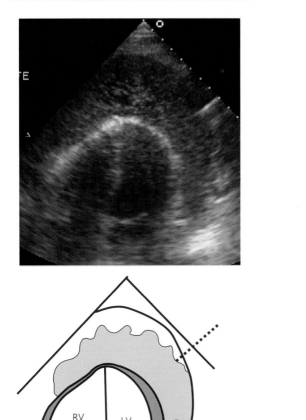

Fig. 8.15 Transthoracic apical echocardiographic view during pericardiocentesis. Agitated saline has been injected down the pericardiocentesis needle to confirm its location within the pericardial space. Bubbles are evident within the pericardial effusion.

Aorta

Aortic atherosclerosis 244
Aortic aneurysm 246
Aortic dissection 248
Intramural haematoma 252
Marfan syndrome 254
Aortic coarctation 256

Aortic atherosclerosis

Aortic atherosclerosis is nearly universal by midlife. Its severity is governed by factors including diabetes, hypercholesterolaemia, hypertension, and smoking. It can be clinically manifested as aneurysms, embolization from atheromatous plaques, obstruction (commonly the infrarenal aorta), and penetration of plaque into the media that can initiate dissection.

Aortic atherosclerosis is a sign of increased cardiovascular risk from coronary artery, cerebrovascular and renovascular disease. Plaques can be identified on transoesophageal echocardiography (TOE) see Fig. 9.1. Calcific plaques are readily visualized on computed tomography and rarely on plane films.

Penetrating atherosclerotic ulcer

- Ulceration of an atherosclerotic lesion of the aorta that penetrates the elastic lamina of the aorta allowing haematoma formation within the media.
- Usually occurs in the descending aorta in elderly smokers.
- Clinical presentation is similar to aortic dissection with chest or back pain.
- In up to 25% of cases, penetration through to the adventitia results in formation of a false aneurysm, and transmural aortic rupture occurs in up to 10% of cases.
- Aortography is the diagnostic standard.
- Standard treatment is high-risk surgery, but there has been increasing success with the use of endovascular stents (Fig. 9.2).

Athero-embolism

- Embolization of plaque material from the luminal surface of a severely diseased aortic segment to cerebral, coronary, visceral, and renal circulations and extremeties is a common cause of mortality and morbidity.
- TOE can identify such material as well as spontaneous contrast.
- Anticoagulation can reduce the risk of future events, as can statin and antiplatelet use.

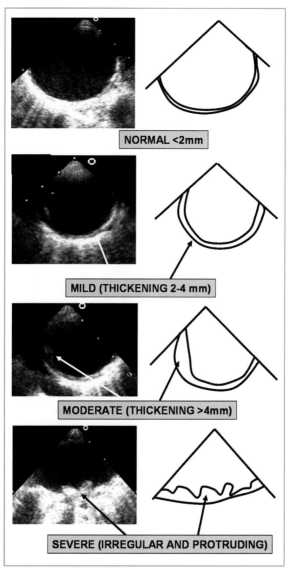

NORMAL <2mm

MILD (THICKENING 2-4 mm)

MODERATE (THICKENING >4mm)

SEVERE (IRREGULAR AND PROTRUDING)

Fig. 9.1 Transoesophageal echocardiography images of atherosclerosis in the descending aorta. The images demonstrate the grades of severity from normal to severe.

Aortic aneurysm

- Commonly seen in the abdominal aorta.
- Degeneration of the media results in widening of the lumen and loss of structural integrity.
- Elastic recoil is lost and ischaemic changes can be precipitated through obstruction of the vasa vasorum.
- Multiple factors, such as genetic defects in collagen, collagenase, and elastase, are believed to be involved in the mechanism resulting in vessel wall injury. Atherosclerosis is thought to contribute to the pathogenesis as a secondary response to vessel wall injury.

Chest X-ray

On plain X-ray aortic wall calcification is seen in less than half of aortic aneurysms, leading to a high false-negative rate. Therefore plain X-ray is not routinely recommended in suspected cases.

Ultrasound (Fig. 9.2)

This is a sensitive test for screening patients at risk of abdominal aortic aneurysms or to monitor size over time. It is of limited value for detecting leakage, rupture, or branch artery involvement

CT

CT is highly sensitive for detecting abdominal aortic aneurysms. It can also detect leakage or rupture and accurately define size and shape, involvement of branch arteries, and adjacent organ involvement. 3D series are used to plan endovascular procedures.

Cardiac magnetic resonance

Imaging of the aorta is equivalent to CT. Advantages are avoidance of dye and superior imaging of branch vessels compared with CT or ultrasound.

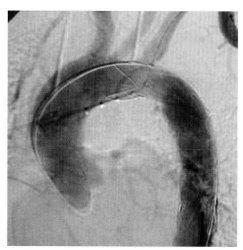

Fig. 9.2 Aortography during implantation of a covered stent in a patient with limited rupture of the descending aorta. The stent is carefully positioned just distal to the left subclavian artery. Reproduced with permission from Myerson SG, Choudhury RP, and Mitchell ARJ (2010) *Emergencies in Cardiology* 2e, Oxford University Press.

Aortic dissection

An aortic dissection is a tear in the aortic intima through which blood enters the aortic wall and strips the media from the adventitia (Fig. 9.3).
- The dissection may result in fatal aortic rupture or propagate distally generating a blood-filled space between the dissected layers.
- The blood supply to major branches (including the coronary arteries) may be compromised.
- If the aortic root is involved, the aortic valve may become incompetent and retrograde propagation to the pericardium may result in cardiac tamponade.

The most common site for aortic dissection is in the proximal ascending aorta within a few centimetres of the aortic valve or in the descending aorta just distal to the left subclavian artery.

Aortic dissection is usually classified according to the Stanford classification (Fig. 9.4), which influences subsequent management:
- type A aortic dissection involves the ascending aorta and management is usually a surgical emergency
- type B aortic dissection spares the ascending aorta and management is initially medical.

Imaging should be performed as quickly as possible using the most accessible and accurate modality available in the hospital. This is usually CT and transthoracic echocardiography. It is important to assess the entry site of the dissection, whether the aortic valve is competent, if there is a pericardial effusion or tamponade, and if there is involvement of the coronary arteries.

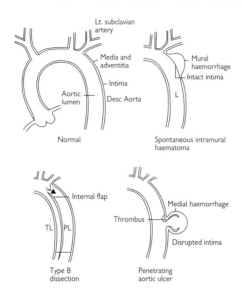

Fig. 9.3 A spontaneous intramural haematoma is characterized by an intact intima with bleeding into the media. Type B aortic dissection usually starts distal to the left subclavian artery. A penetrating aortic ulcer involves a disrupted intima and haemorrhage into the media. Reproduced with permission from Myerson SG, Choudhury RP, and Mitchell ARJ (2010) *Emergencies in Cardiology* 2e, Oxford University Press.

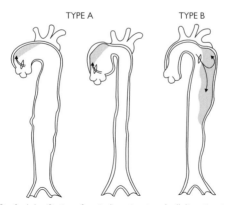

Fig. 9.4 Stanford classification of aortic dissection: type A, all dissections involving the ascending aorta; type B, dissections not involving the ascending aorta. Reproduced with permission from Myerson SG, Choudhury RP, and Mitchell ARJ (2010) *Emergencies in Cardiology* 2e, Oxford University Press.

Chest X-ray (Fig. 9.5)

- An abnormal aortic silhouette appears in up to 90% of cases (NB 10% of chest X-rays will appear normal).
- Separation of the intimal calcification that occurs in the aortic knob by more than 1cm (the 'calcium sign') is suggestive of aortic dissection.
- Left-sided pleural effusions may occur and are more common with descending dissections

CT

With modern spiral scanners, this has a sensitivity and specificity of 96–100% and is the standard investigation for suspected aortic dissection.

Cardiac magnetic resonance

- Sensitivity and specificity of nearly 100%
- Non-invasive
- Availability and reduced access to an unwell patient are the main limitations on its use.

Transoesophageal echocardiography (Fig. 9.6)

- Useful for imaging the proximal ascending aorta, identifying involvement of coronary ostia, and examining the aortic valve.
- Sensitivity of ~98% and specificity of ~95%.
- Patients usually require sedation.
- Ideally performed immediately prior to surgery after surgical consent has been obtained.

Transthoracic echocardiography

- Can determine the involvement of the aortic valve, determine left ventricular function, and identify pericardial effusions.
- Sensitivity of 59–85% and specificity of 63–96%.
- A normal transthoracic echocardiogram does not exclude aortic dissection.

Aortography

- Invasive procedure with associated risks.
- Requires contrast material and takes time to perform.
- Sensitivity of 77–88% and specificity of 94%.
- It is now rarely performed as other imaging techniques are quicker and safer.

Coronary angiography

Not routinely performed in patients with aortic dissection. Chronic coronary disease is seen in a quarter of patients with aortic dissection, but this has not been shown to have a significant impact on outcome.

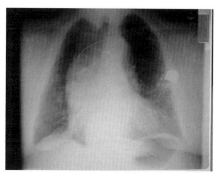

Fig. 9.5 Chest X-ray in a patient with a large ascending aortic aneurysm and a type A aortic dissection. The pacemaker wire is displaced laterally by the size of the aorta.

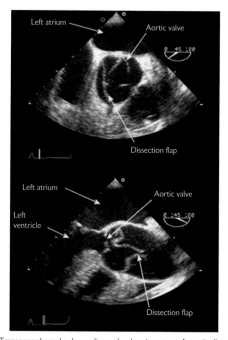

Fig. 9.6 Transoesophageal echocardiography showing a type A aortic dissection. There is a dissection flap just above the aortic valve in the proximal ascending aorta. Top: transverse view. Bottom: longitudinal view. Reproduced with permission from Myerson SG, Choudhury RP, and Mitchell ARJ (2010) *Emergencies in Cardiology* 2e, Oxford University Press.

Intramural haematoma

- The result of haemorrhage within the media and adventitia of the aortic wall.
- The aortic intima remains intact.
- Believed to be due to rupture of the aortic vasa vasorum.
- Presentation can mimic aortic dissection.
- Patients are typically elderly with a history of hypertension, and many have aortic atherosclerosis.
- There is increasing evidence that an intramural haematoma may be a precursor of aortic dissection.
- Treat as for aortic dissection with analgesia and intravenous anti-hypertensive agents.
- Surgery is indicated when the ascending aorta is involved.

CT and cardiac magnetic resonance (Figs. 9.7 and 9.8)

- CT or CMR imaging are the investigations of choice.
- The diagnosis is made by excluding an intimal tear.
- A non-contrast-enhancing crescent along the aortic wall with no false lumen or associated atherosclerotic ulcer is usually demonstrated.

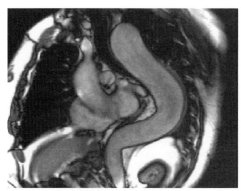

Fig. 9.7 CMR image of an intramural haematoma in the descending thoracic aorta.

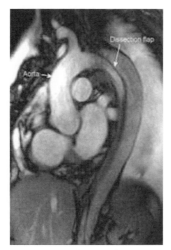

Fig. 9.8 CMR image of a type B aortic dissection. There is a dissection flap in the descending aorta. Reproduced with permission from Myerson SG, Choudhury RP, and Mitchell ARJ (2010) *Emergencies in Cardiology 2e*, Oxford University Press.

Marfan syndrome

- Autosomal dominant connective tissue disease with a prevalence of at least 1:10000.
- Common cardiovascular features are:
  - mitral valve prolapse (75%).
  - dilatation of the aortic sinuses (90%).
- Aortic dilatation is usually limited to the proximal ascending aorta with loss of the sinotubular junction and a flask-shaped appearance (Fig. 9.9).
- Aortic regurgitation is common when the aorta reaches 50mm in diameter (normal diameter <40mm).
- The risk of dissection increases with the diameter of the aorta but occurs relatively infrequently at diameters <55mm.
- Aortic dissection in Marfan syndrome is usually type A and begins just above the coronary ostia. 10% of cases begin distal to the left subclavian artery (type B).

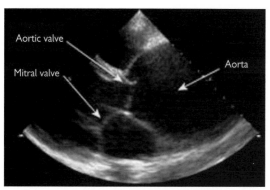

Fig. 9.9 Transthoracic echocardiography of an enlarged ascending aorta in a patient with Marfan syndrome. Reproduced with permission from Myerson SG, Choudhury RP, and Mitchell ARJ (2010) *Emergencies in Cardiology 2e*, Oxford University Press.

Aortic coarctation

Aortic coarctation is a narrowing of the aorta in the region of the ligamentum arteriosum, just distal to the left subclavian artery, see p. 278. If severe, the lower body relies on collateral vessels via the intercostal arteries for perfusion. Complete occlusion is also possible. A 'simple' coarctation is one without other cardiac lesions. A 'complex' coarctation is associated with other defects such as a ventricular septal defect or left-sided obstructive lesion (e.g. aortic stenosis). At least 50% of patients with aortic coarctation have a bicuspid aortic valve. The clinical signs that can be present include the following.

- Upper limb hypertension and differential arm–leg pulses. Blood pressure measurement in the right arm and a leg is necessary in all new patients with hypertension. A pressure difference of ≥30mmHg may suggest coarctation.
- Continuous murmur in the interscapular region.

Chest X-ray

- 'Three sign' caused by narrowing of the aorta at the site of coarctation with dilatation of the vessel before and after the coarctation.
- 'Rib notching' caused by erosions of the inferior edge of the ribs by enlarged intercostal arteries.

Cardiac CT

Good visualization of location and severity using contrast and reconstructed images.

Cardiac magnetic resonance

Excellent visualization of anatomy, possible aneurysm formation, and, using contrast angiography, 3D visualization of the geometry and collaterals (Fig. 9.10). Velocity measurements can assess the degree of stenosis.

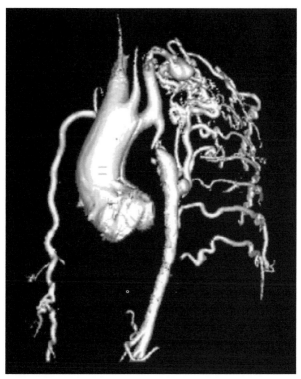

Fig. 9.10 3D volume rendered CMR image of a coarctation with multiple collaterals demonstrated.

Congenital heart disease

Congenital heart disease 260
Chest X-ray 262
Echocardiography 264
Transoesophageal echocardiography 266
Cardiac magnetic resonance 268
Cardiac CT 270
Cardiac catheterization 272
Atrial and ventricular septal defects 274
Aortic coarctation 276
Transposition of the great arteries 278
Tetralogy of Fallot 280
Aberrant coronary anatomy 282
Patent ductus arteriosus 282
Major aorto-pulmonary collateral arteries (MAPCAs) 282
Pulmonary arterial hypertension including
    Eisenmenger's syndrome 284

Congenital heart disease

The phrase 'congenital heart disease' encompasses a range of cardio-vascular problems from simple patent foramen ovale (PFO) to complex conditions such as tetralogy of Fallot. Cardiovascular imaging is essential in the diagnosis and understanding of congenital heart disease. Many specialists who train in congenital heart disease include a dedicated imaging component in their training.

Cardiovascular imaging

- CMR and transthoracic echocardiography (TTE) are the modalities of choice for the routine assessment and follow-up of patients with congenital heart disease.
- TTE is fundamental to the assessment of congenital heart disease, particularly in the acute setting and at initial diagnosis, but requires a high level of expertise.
- All major centres for congenital heart disease will have access to CMR although studies are time-consuming (30–60min) and any patient with a pacemaker or an implantable cardioverter defibrillator (ICD) is currently excluded from CMR examination.
- CT has been used in the assessment of congenital heart disease for many years, but predominantly for non-cardiac indications such as CT pulmonary angiography. Any patient who is unable or unwilling to undergo CMR can be assessed by multi-detector CT (MDCT). Although flow data will not be available, most other aspects of a CMR study are available within the MDCT dataset.

Chest X-ray

Advantages of chest X-ray
• Widely available
• Allows serial comparison

Disadvantages of chest X-ray
• Limited data on intracardiac anatomy
• Two-dimensional with compression of 3D data

What can chest X-ray tell us?
An important point to check in congenital heart disease is the left and right labels on the CXR! In a normal chest X-ray there will be a left fundal bubble, a left cardiac apex, long left and short right bronchi, and a right-sided liver. Some key signs of congenital heart disease to be aware of are the following.
• Situs: fundal bubble (usually left); cardiac apex (usually left), bronchial tree (normally long left, short right), position of liver (Fig. 10.1).
• Extracardiac: trachea, cervical ribs, thoracotomy/sternotomy scars, kyphoscoliosis, diaphragms? Raised post-op, clips, prosthetic devices, sternal wires (not always used in paediatric cardiac surgery), pacemaker/ICDs and position of leads, rib notching in aortic coarctation (Fig. 10.2).
• Cardiothoracic ratio:?enlarged,?dilated right-side.
• Cardiac silhouette: certain typical patterns.
• Aortic arch:?collaterals, right-sided arch.
• Calcification of conduits.
• Pulmonary arteries: dilatation or absence.
• Lung markings: vascular and parenchyma.
• Pleural effusions.

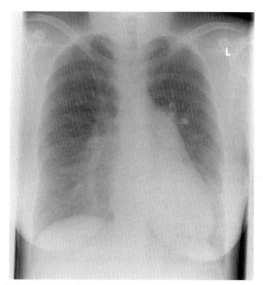

Fig. 10.1 30-year-old female patient with an unoperated secundum atrial septal defect showing dilated right heart, enlarged pulmonary arteries, and pulmonary plethora.

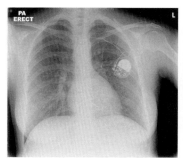 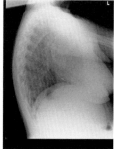

Fig. 10.2 29-year-old female patient with transposition of the great arteries with a stent in the superior baffle and a ventricular pacing lead through the stent into the subpulmonary left ventricle.

Echocardiography

Advantages of echocardiography
- Portable and widely used non-invasive imaging tool
- Non-invasive detailed anatomical information with serial assessment
- Flow assessment.

Disadvantages of echocardiography
- Anatomical knowledge and understanding of congenital heart disease essential when performing echoes
- Studies are operator dependent
- May be difficult to see some aspects of the cardiac system or vascular connection.

What can echocardiography tell us?
All the basic principles of TTE (assessment of ventricular function, valvular function, and presence of a pericardial effusion) are usually possible in all patients and a full dataset is acquired, including suprasternal, subcostal, and right parasternal views (Figs. 10.3 and 10.4). Some key aspects that are of importance when performing echocardiography in congenital heart disease patients are as follows.
- It is useful to start imaging after you have tried to visualize the anatomy.
- A sequential segmental approach must be used in all patients.
- Patients may have more than one lesion.
- Doppler assessment of valves, aortic arch (coarctation), shunt calculation (rarely used), and baffle obstruction (patients who have had arterial switch transposition of the great arteries (TGA)) is possible.
- Contrast bubble echo can be used for the identification of shunts (e.g. PFO).
- Dobutamine stress echo can be used in patients who have had arterial switch TGA to assess for ischaemia.
- Advanced techniques can all be used to derive further information, including tissue Doppler for ventricular function and 3D for detailed anatomical information (e.g. Ebstein's anomaly, atrioventricular septal defect), speckle tracking, and dyssynchrony assessment.

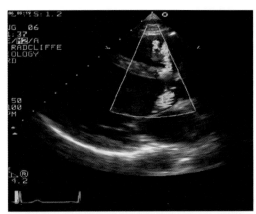

Fig. 10.3 Parasternal long-axis view with TTE demonstrating a perimembranous ventricular septal defect (VSD). Colour flow mapping shows the jet between the left ventricular outflow tract and the right ventricle. In this situation it is important to assess the aortic valve and identify any aortic regurgitation.

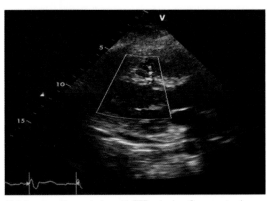

Fig. 10.4 Parasternal long-axis view with TTE and colour flow mapping demonstrating a muscular VSD. There may be multiple defects and therefore the colour Doppler must be placed along the whole length of the ventricular septum during the study.

Transoesophageal echocardiography

What can TOE tell us?

Experience is essential for interpreting TOE in complex CHD and therefore should be undertaken in specialist centres and/or by specialists in congenital heart disease. TOE is usually used perioperatively to assess patients before and during the procedure. This is the case for both surgical and percutaneous procedures (ASD/PFO/VSD closure, valve surgery) (Fig. 10.5). Increasingly 3D TOE is being used to allow better visualization of variation in the 3D cardiac anatomy.

Two things to be aware of in patients with congenital heart disease are as follows:

- care should be taken with sedation as this may result in cardiovascular collapse
- always check for previous oesophageal surgery or abnormalities.

A sequential analysis is used and some of the particular areas of the cardiovascular system that lend themselves to evaluation by TOE are:

- pulmonary veins
- pathways/baffles/communications/intracardiac thrombus (prior to cardioversion)
- contrast/bubble echo to identify shunts/PFO
- assessment of endocarditis
- assessments of aorta such as patent ductus arteriosus (PDA), coarctation, outflow tract obstruction
- patients with difficult transthoracic views (e.g. chest deformity)
- ventricular function from transgastric views in patients with difficult views.

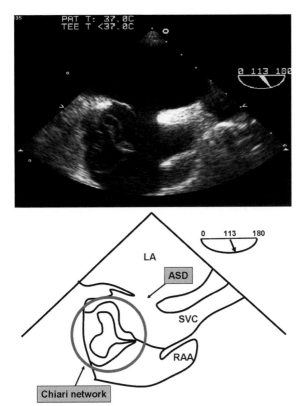

Fig. 10.5 Transoesophageal bicaval view demonstrating a secundum atrial septal defect. A Chiari network with multiple stands of the network extending across the right atrium is also evident.

Cardiac magnetic resonance

Advantages of CMR
- Any imaging plane is possible.
- Independent of body habitus.
- Accurate quantification of cardiac chambers.
- Can assess vasculature and aorta as well as heart.
- Can study chest and other areas of body during the same study.

Disadvantages of CMR
- Specialist experience in both congenital heart disease and CMR are essential during acquisition (to ensure that the correct sequences are recorded) and interpretation scan. Therefore congenital CMRs are usually only undertaken in specialist centres.
- Expensive and limited availability.
- Potentially lengthy scans with long breath-holds.
- Susceptibility to artefacts from stents, sternal wires, and rods from spinal deformity surgery.
- Pacemakers, ICDS, metallic implants, and aneurysm clips are contraindicated.
- Some patients are claustrophobic (2%).

What can CMR tell us?
CMR is a standard cardiovascular investigation for assessment of congenital heart disease. It is particularly useful for the following.
- Non-invasive detailed anatomy and communications: assessment of anaomalous branches (e.g. anomalous pulmonary veins), connections, and collaterals; assessment of pre- and post-surgery anatomy (Fig. 10.6).
- Accurate quantification of left and right ventricular volumes, mass, and function. Excellent serial follow-up.
- Accurate quantification of valvular and sub- or supravalvular disease, severity of stenosis, and regurgitation. Excellent assessment of aortic coarctation repair and identification of aneurysms and re-coarctation.
- Assessment of flow and quantification of shunts.
- Assessment of suitability for percutaneous closure of atrial septal defects.
- Assessment of scar, fibrosis, and thrombus with intravenous contrast imaging.
- Identification of surgical or interventional complications.

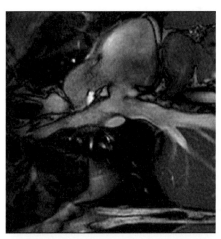

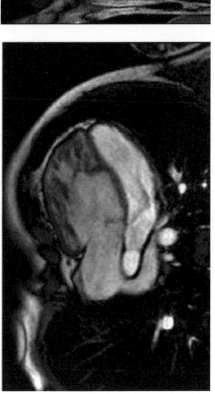

Fig. 10.6 CMR of a patient with transposition of the great arteries. The patient has had an atrial switch and patent baffles are evident.

Cardiac CT

Advantages of cardiac CT
- Rapid data acquisition.
- Whole-heart dataset collected for post-processing.
- Extracardiac anatomy can be assessed.
- Suitable for those unwilling or unable to undergo CMR.

Disadvantages of cardiac CT
- Specialist experience in both congenital heart disease and cardiac CT is essential: Therefore congenital cardiac CT is usually only undertaken in specialist congenital centres
- Susceptibility artefacts from stents, sternal wires, and rods from spinal deformity surgery
- Ionizing radiation dose makes sequential analysis unattractive
- Patient selection is important as multiphase reformatting of MDCT data utilizes retrospective gating techniques and therefore a stable heart rhythm is required.

What can cardiac CT tell us?
Traditional indications such as CT pulmonary angiography (CTPA) in the assessment of pulmonary hypertension and the imaging of extra-cardiac structures remain frequent indications for CT, but the ability to combine these studies with those of CT coronary angiography, ventricular function analysis, and valvular assessment mean that the indications for cardiac MDCT in the congenital heart disease population are wide. Although flow data are not available, most other aspects of a CMR study can be obtained from the MDCT dataset. Application of basic principles of sequential analysis and imaging techniques should be used in interpretation.

- MDCT delivers accurate assessment of gross morphological cardiac, coronary, and great cardiac vessel anatomy, allowing most congenital malformations to be delineated (Fig. 10.7).
- Non-invasive detailed anatomy and communications: assessment of anomalous branches (e.g. anomalous pulmonary veins), connections, and collaterals, and assessment of pre- and post-surgery anatomy are all possible with cardiac CT.
- Accurate quantification of left ventricular volumes, mass, and function is possible with standard CT coronary angiogram protocols. RV assessment is possible with extended protocols.

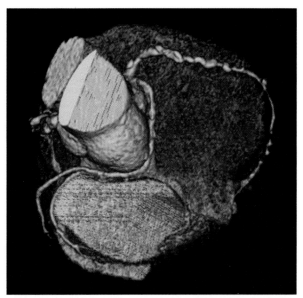

Fig. 10.7 Aberrant left circumflex artery off calcified right coronary artery demonstrated with cardiac CT.

Cardiac catheterization

What can cardiac catheterization tell us?

Cardiac catheterization provides an opportunity for both imaging and pressure data collection (including pulmonary artery pressure and pulmonary vascular resistance). Therefore both left and right heart catheterizations are usually performed and a full study (including saturations, pressures and angiograms) is acquired.

- Essential haemodynamic measures include:
  - saturations: IVC, SVC, PA, femoral artery (RA/RV/LV/PV)
  - mixed venous saturations: $(3 \times SVC + IVC)/4$
  - Qp:Qs = (Ao saturation − mixed venous saturations)/(PV saturation − PA saturation).
  - pressure measurements: RA (a wave, v wave and mean), RV (systolic, diastolic, and mean), PA (systolic, diastolic, and mean; left and right), PCWP (a wave, v wave and mean).
  - femoral artery (systolic, diastolic, and mean), aorta (systolic, diastolic, and mean), and LV (systolic, diastolic, and mean).
- Angiography (use biplane if possible): assess LV and RV function, outflow tracts, ventricular septum, atrioventricular valves, aortograms, pulmonary arteriography, and coronary angiography.
- Incidental congenital lesions may be identified at catheterization (e.g. IVC interruption, aortic coarctation, anomalous coronary arteries, PFO/ASD, coronary fistulas).

Right heart catheterization in patients with adult congenital heart disease requires a high level of expertise because of the altered anatomy. Previous angiograms/intervention/cutdowns may also make femoral access difficult. Because of the level of expertise needed for interpretation and data collection studies are ideally performed at specialist adult congenital heart disease centres.

Atrial and ventricular septal defects

Intracardiac shunts should be suspected in any patient with a dilated right heart and the septa should be imaged. The usual modality of choice for the septa, particularly the atrial septum, is TOE. TOE may characterize defects in the ventricular septum or further modalities may be required. The following features are assessed in imaging:

- right heart size and function
- identification of pulmonary veins
- coexistent mitral valve disease
- size of defect and presence of rims, and hence suitability for percutaneous closure (secundum)
- pulmonary artery pressure
- LV function
- other lesions (e.g. Ebstein's anomaly, VSD).

Echocardiography

- TTE may allow initial identification of ASDs and VSDs (Fig. 10.8). However, TOE is required to characterize the defect.
- TOE is good for identification of the pulmonary veins (?anomalous RUPV,?sinus venosus ASD).
- Primum ASD is the atrial component of an atrioventricular septal defect (loss of normal 'offsetting' of AV valves) and therefore it is important to assess for AV valve regurgitation, LVOT obstruciton, VSD component, and pulmonary vascular disease.
- Intraprocedural TOE, can be useful to guide closure of defects.

Angiography

- Shunt calculation, coronary angiography (prior to surgical repair), pulmonary venous drainage.
- Percutaneous closure at same procedure.

Cardiac magnetic resonance

- Detailed anatomy and accurate quantification of right/left heart volumes and function.
- Identification of pulmonary veins.
- Coexistent mitral valve disease
- Size of defect and presence of rims, and hence suitability for percutaneous closure (secundum ASD and some VSDs).
- Shunt quantification (Qp:Qs) from pulmonary artery and aortic flow.

Cardiac CT

- Characterization of defect (i.e. location and size) (Fig. 10.9).
- Biventricular dimensions and function.
- Associated anomalies such as anomalous pulmonary venous drainage can be readily visualized.
- Cardiac CT can also be used to follow up patients after surgical or percutaneous ASD closure, evaluating RV function or the state of a septal occlusion device.
- The 3D capabilities of CCT allow detailed anatomic information about features of a PFO)and VSD size and location.

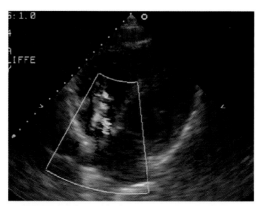

Fig. 10.8 TTE subcostal view with colour flow mapping placed across the atrial septum to demonstrate a secundum ASD.

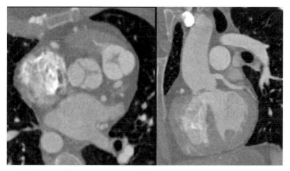

Fig. 10.9 Cardiac CT axial and sagittal views of a patient with a common arterial trunk. A VSD is evident on the saggital view (white arrow).

Aortic coarctation

Aortic coarctation requires imaging to determine the severity of disease, impact on the heart, and associated disease (bicuspid aortic valve, Turners syndrome) and to allow serial follow-up after intervention on the coarctation.

Echocardiography

Echocardiography can be used to measure LV hypertrophy and LV function, and to identify if there is evidence of a bicuspid aortic valve or coexistent aortic valve disease. Suprasternal views will also allow assessment of dilated ascending or descending aorta (Turner's syndrome),? re-coarctation, or aneurysm. Further imaging with CMR or cardiac CT is usually required.

Cardiac magnetic resonance

- Formal quantification of LV mass.
- ?Left ventricular hypertrophy if associated bicuspid aortic valve (85%), subaortic or aortic valve disease.
- Accurate quantification of LV volumes and function.
- Accurate visualization of dilated ascending or descending aorta (Turner's syndrome),?re-coarctation, aneurysm or dissection (Fig. 10.10).
- Dilated or anomalous head and neck vessels
- If aortic coarctation stent, patient will need CT to assess for stent fracture or complications of the intervention because of imaging artefacts.

Cardiac CT

- Location and severity of aortic coarctation: isotropic voxels allow the selection of any desired imaging plane after acquisition. May be particularly useful for isthmic coarctation.
- Re-coarctation, aneurysm, or dissection: CCT is better than CMR and TTE for assessing stent patency after percutaneous treatment (Fig. 10.11). Thus may be valuable in both the diagnosis and follow-up of these patients, i.e. where stent fracture is suspected.
- LV mass, volumes, and function can be obtained.
- Vascular assessment can include imaging to look for dilatation of ascending/descending aorta and anomalous head and neck vessels.

Angiography

Information on coarctation can be obtained at angiography and is used for percutaneous interventions on the coarctation. Usual procedure is:
- aortogram (RAO and lateral projections)
- coronary angiography (patients may have chest pain)
- LV angiogram with pullback across aortic valve (80% bicuspid aortic valve)
- measurement of gradient across coarctation (care when crossing coarctation or repair site)
- percutaneous balloon/stent at same procedure.

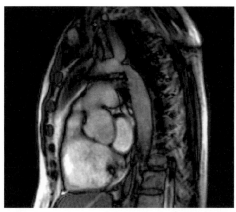

Fig. 10.10 CMR oblique sagittal plane optimized to pass through a native co-arctation.

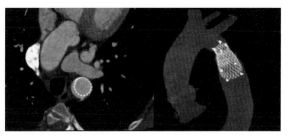

Fig. 10.11 Cardiac CT axial and sagittal views of a coarctation stent.

Transposition of the great arteries

Following initial diagnosis, ongoing imaging of patients with transposition of the great arteries needs to be optimized to monitor surgical repair. The likely repairs include an atrial switch (Mustard or Senning) and (from the late 1980s) an arterial switch. The Fontan circulation describes the creation of a cavopulmonary connection, the patency of which is crucial to maintain pulmonary blood flow. Echocardiography may be useful to monitor flow in baffles, particularly with TOE, but full assessment of patients will usually require CMR or cardiac CT.

Echocardiography

Atrial switch

Echocardiography can be used to assess the following.

- Systemic RV function (including tricuspid annular plane systolic excursion (TAPSE), TDI).
- Systemic AV valve regurgitation (tricuspid valve).
- Baffle leak or obstruction (colour and PW Doppler): normal <1.5m/s with good arterial Doppler signal; sniff test, <100% IVC collapse suggests inferior baffle obstruction.
- subpulmonary LV function.

Arterial switch

LV and RV function (any regional wall motion abnormality (RWMA)), aortic root dilatation or aortic regurgitation, coronary ostia, pulmonary valve/arteries (?stenosis).

Fontan

Sequential analysis, ventricular function, AV valve regurgitation, patent pathway (IVC and SVC connections),?thrombus formation.

Cardiac magnetic resonance (Fig. 10.12)

Atrial switch

Quantification of systemic RV function and subpulmonary LV function and systemic AV valve regurgitation (tricuspid valve).

Arterial switch

CMR will provide information on the following.

- LV and RV volumes, mass, and function (any RWMA).
- Aortic root dilatation or aortic regurgitation.
- Coronary ostia.
- Pulmonary valve/arteries (?stenosis, particularly if LeCompte manoeuvre). Evidence of scar or previous subendocardial infarction with contrast imaging.

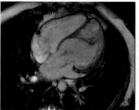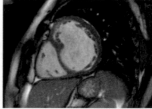

Fig. 10.12 CMR long- and short-axis images of a patient with congenitally corrected transposition of the great arteries. Note the dilated and trabeculated (with moderator band) systemic right ventricle with tricuspid (systemic AV valve) regurgitation.

Cardiac CT

Cardiac CT can confirm atrioventricular and ventriculo-arterial discordance and evaluate any anatomical repair, including biventricular size and function.

Atrial switch

Patency of intra-atrial baffles or ventriculo-arterial conduits (Rastelli procedure).

Arterial switch

Monitor neo-aortic and neo-pulmonary arteries. In the latter case, the ostia of coronary arteries are re-implanted into the neo-aorta and may be assessed.

Fontan circulation

- Readily visualized using 3D reconstruction techniques.
- Abnormal vessel dimensions, stenoses and post-stenotic dilatation, mural damage (such as dissection or calcification) and *in situ* thrombosis.
- Right atrial size and pulmonary venous return are also assessed.

Common arterial trunk

The value of cardiac CT in patients with truncal abnormalities is well established. Intravenous contrast allows identification of pulmonary artery branches and collaterals, where present. In those who have undergone surgical repair, cardiac CT is able to assess conduit patency accurately.

Tetralogy of Fallot

Tetralogy of Fallot can have complex anatomy and corrective surgery. Echocardiography provides a useful first-line investigation to provide haemodynamic parameters, but further imaging is often needed to provide a comprehensive evaluation.

Echocardiography

The key aspects of cardiac anatomy recorded with echocardiography are:
- right ventricular size and function (including TAPSE and RV TDI)
- pulmonary valve/RVOT size (?suitability for percutaneous PVR)
- severity of pulmonary regurgitation (colour, CW Doppler)
- branch pulmonary arteries
- LV size, function and septal dyssynchrony (including Simpson's method, mitral annular plane systolic excursion (MAPSE), TDI lateral and septum),? residual VSD
- tricuspid regurgitation
- LVOT obstruction, dilated aortic root or aortic regurgitation.

Cardiac magnetic resonance

CMR allows precise assessment without limitation of imaging plane and therefore can be used to obtain information on the following.
- Accurate and reproducible RV and LV volumes and function.
- Detailed anatomy of previous repair, including previous shunts and evidence of residual VSD,?dilatation from previous transannular patch
- Evidence of dilated aortic root, LVOT obstruction.
- Evidence of proximal pulmonary artery stenoses, pulmonary valve/ RVOT size (measure suitability for percutaneous PVR) (Fig. 10.13).
- Flow measurement of severity of pulmonary regurgitation (regurgitant volume and fraction), branch pulmonary arteries and flow.
- Other valvular regurgitation including tricuspid and aortic.

Cardiac CT

Cardiac CT allows detailed assessment of intracardiac anatomy and the coronary and pulmonary arteries. It can be used for the following.
- Assessment of previous repair including shunts and valved conduits.
- Assessment of spatial relationship of valves with other cardiac and non-cardiac structures prior to percutaneous procedures, e.g. path of an aberrant coronary artery between conduit and adjacent epicardium (expansion of a stented pulmonary valve may potentially lead to compression of the underlying aberrant coronary artery).

Angiography

During angiography it is possible to collect data on RV function, pulmonary arteries, RVOT with degree of pulmonary regurgitation, residual VSD, and coronary arteries (origins and disease in older patients) (Fig. 10.14).

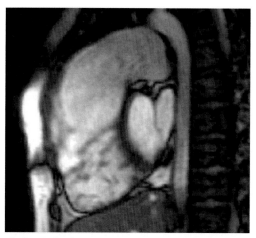

Fig. 10.13 Grossly dilated right ventricular outflow tract demonstrated with CMR in a patient with a transannular repair of tetralogy of Fallot.

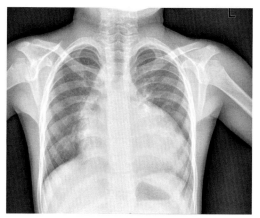

Fig. 10.14 A young boy with previous repair of tetralogy of Fallot with a calcified RVOT conduit and increased cardiothoracic ratio from severe pulmonary regurgitation and dilated right heart.

Aberrant coronary anatomy

Because of the high incidence of abnormal resting ECGs, exercise testing is often unhelpful in those with adult congenital heart disease. Invasive coronary angiography can be effective in identification of anomalous coronaries, although it may be technically challenging. There is also often no evidence of obstructive coronary artery disease on invasive angiography. CTA (CT coronary angiography) offers excellent negative predictive value for the exclusion of coronary artery disease and is a powerful alternative to invasive coronary angiography in this setting. CTA is helpful in assessing the origin and course of anomalous coronary arteries which are seen frequently in those with abnormal cardiovascular anatomy. CTA is also useful in patients with Kawasaki's disease, where the site, size, and number of coronary artery aneurysms can be measured, as can the extent of calcification, thrombus, and contrast enhancement within any aneurysms seen. CCT is also a well-established technique for identifying and fully delineating coronary fistulas and venous anatomy. Increasingly, CMR is able to provide information on coronary anatomy, particularly of the proximal coronaries. Echocardiography has been used for serial monitoring of coronaries in patients following Kawasaki's disease, but does not provide definitive information on coronary anatomy.

Patent ductus arteriosus

- Patent ductus arteriosus (PDA) is occasionally found incidentally on CT acquisitions, particularly during investigation of pulmonary arterial hypertension (PAH).
- Cardiac CT and CMR can accurately determine the presence and size of a PDA and, with the use of 3D reconstruction techniques, provide accurate images for surgical correction where necessary (Fig. 10.15).
- Cardiac CT is also able to quantify calcification within the duct. Heavy PDA calcification is associated with a higher surgical risk and may result in referral for trans-catheter closure or aortic stenting, rather than surgery.

Major aorto-pulmonary collateral arteries (MAPCAs)

MAPCAs develop in conditions such as pulmonary atresia when blood fails to reach the lungs via the pulmonary arteries. The anatomy of these collateral arteries varies widely, and accurate delineation is crucial to clinical management. The high 3D spatial resolution offered by cardiac CT and CMR lends itself to accurate anatomical localization and may usefully guide interventional or surgical management (Fig. 10.16).

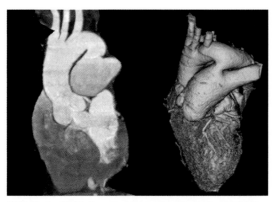

Fig. 10.15 Cardiac CT 2D slice and volume-rendered image of a patent ductus arteriosus.

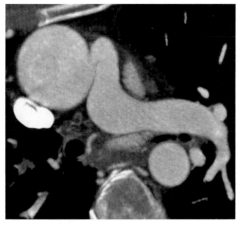

Fig. 10.16 Axial cardiac CT image of main pulmonary artery arising from ascending aorta.

Pulmonary arterial hypertension including Eisenmenger's syndrome

CT pulmonary angiography (CTPA) has been the mainstay of diagnostic imaging in pulmonary arterial hypertension (PAH) for many years. CTPA allows:

- identification or exclusion of thrombo-embolic disease
- delineation of confluence and size of the pulmonary arteries and any inherent stenoses or aneurysmal dilatation of these vessels.

CT coronary angiography in conjunction with standard CTPA allows:

- evaluation of RV hypertrophy
- evaluation of biventricular function
- differentiation of intrinsic and extrinsic pulmonary arterial pathology.

Although flow and pressure measurements are not possible with cardiac CT, the aetiologies underlying Eisenmenger's syndrome, valve integrity, and biventricular function can be readily assessed.

Arrhythmias

Arrhythmias *286*
Atrial arrhythmias *288*
Supraventricular tachycardia *290*
Ventricular tachycardia *292*
Ventricular fibrillation *294*
Cardiac arrest *294*
Arrhythmogenic right ventricular cardiomyopathy (ARVC) *294*
Catheter ablation of arrhythmias *296*

Arrhythmias

Background
Cardiac imaging is an important part of the investigation of patients with cardiac arrhythmia. There are many structural cardiac conditions that can predispose to the development of cardiac rhythm problems. As treatment moves away from long-term medication to curative catheter ablation, information from echocardiography, computed tomography (CT) and cardiac magnetic resonance (CMR) are increasingly being used to plan as well as guide procedures.

Palpitation
'Palpitation' is defined as a patient's awareness of an abnormal heartbeat. A combination of history, physical examination, surface 12-lead ECGs, and ambulatory ECGs is usually adequate to make a diagnosis. It is important to establish whether the symptoms are a result of structural heart disease. For this reason, transthoracic echocardiography is central in the diagnostic algorithm. Abnormalities of left ventricular size and function can be seen. Left atrial enlargement is common in patients with atrial fibrillation (AF). Occasionally CMR is required for further structural assessment of the myocardium in suspected cardiomyopathy.

Syncope
Syncope is 'A transient, self-limited sudden loss of consciousness, usually leading to falling'. Syncope can be caused by a wide spectrum of conditions, ranging from the benign faint to potentially fatal cardiac arrhythmias. Imaging is guided by the clinical history and examination findings. For example, a patient with a systolic murmur may require transthoracic echocardiography to exclude aortic stenosis or hypertrophic cardiomyopathy. A patient presenting with syncope and unequal blood pressures in the upper limbs may have aortic dissection, and cross-sectional imaging might be considered.

Atrial arrhythmias

An understanding of the mechanism by which atrial tachyarrhythmias are initiated and sustained is important in developing strategies to plan and perform catheter ablation procedures. Arrhythmias involving the atria can be divided into those contained completely in the atria and those requiring activation of both the atrium and ventricle.

Atrial tachycardia

Atrial focus of cells firing faster than the sinoatrial node. Catheter ablation can offer a cure in symptomatic drug-refractory cases.

Atrial flutter

Typically there is a re-entry circuit within the right atrium which can be interrupted by ablating a series of lesions, creating a conduction block between the inferior vena cava and tricuspid valve. Re-entry circuits may also be found in the left atrium.

Atrial fibrillation (Figs. 11.1 and 11.2)

AF is the most common cardiac arrhythmia, affecting 1% of the population. There is chaotic electrical activation of the atria resulting in loss of coordinated contractile function. This can be from a single focus of cells with enhanced automaticity or from a single or several micro-re-entry circuits that depolarize rapidly, creating self-perpetuating waves of electrical activity with variable conduction resulting in fibrillation. AF ablation strategies are targeted at electrically isolating the four pulmonary veins from the left atrium. These are required to sustain the multiple re-entry circuits that lead to AF. Electrical signals in the superior vena cava and coronary sinus are additional targets.

Cardiovascular imaging

Atrial arrhythmias often occur in patients with structurally normal hearts, but echocardiography should be arranged to exclude underlying cardiomyopathy and to examine valvular function and atrial size. Further imaging is then planned based on findings of additional pathology.

AF can be associated with pulmonary conditions such as pulmonary embolism and pneumonia, and therefore additional imaging of the lungs with chest X-ray or CT may be required if clinically suspected.

In patients presenting with AF in whom electrical cardioversion is being considered, a transoesophageal echocardiogram can help to exclude a left atrial appendage thrombus.

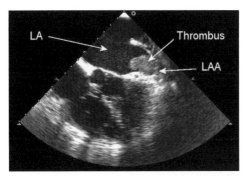

Fig. 11.1 Transoesophageal echocardiogram of the left atrium (LA) demonstrating a thrombus in the left atrial appendage (LAA). It is believed that >90% of strokes in AF result from emboli originating in the LAA.

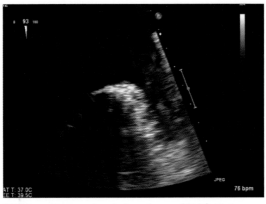

Fig. 11.2 Zoomed transoesophageal echocardiogram of the left atrium demonstrating spontaneous contrast or 'smoke' from the left atrial appendage. This is a marker of high risk for appendage thrombus as it signifies low blood velocities.

Supraventricular tachycardia

Atrioventricular re-entry tachycardia (AVRT)

- Usually requires the AV node and at least one accessory pathway (AP) between the atrium and the ventricle to set up a re-entry circuit, or two accessory pathways without the participation of the AV node.
- Where there is evidence of pre-excitation caused by an AP on the resting ECG, i.e. a short P–R interval and delta wave, the patient is said to have a Wolffe–Parkinson–White (WPW) abnormality. If the patient develops AVRT, they are said to have WPW syndrome.
- Patients with AVRT due to an AP that only conducts retrograde are said to have a concealed pathway, as there is no evidence of it on the resting ECG.
- Catheter ablation of the AP offers a cure for AVRT.

Atrioventricular nodal re-entry tachycardia (AVNRT)

- Re-entry circuit is contained entirely within the AV node.
- Dual conduction pathways within the AV node, typically a slow and fast pathway, allow electrical impulses to recycle and sustain the arrhythmia.
- In drug refractory or intolerant cases catheter ablation offers a cure.

Cardiovascular imaging

- Cardiovascular imaging in these conditions is usually centred on transthoracic echocardiography. This allows exclusion of underlying structural abnormalities, particularly Ebstein's anomaly and hyper trophic cardiomyopathy (Fig. 11.3).
- If myocardial pathology is identified, further imaging with CMR may be required.

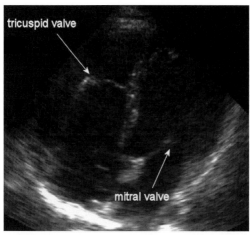

Fig. 11.3 Transthoracic echocardiogram of a patient with Ebstein's anomaly. Compared with the mitral valve the leaflets of the tricuspid valve are displaced towards the apex of the heart. This can be associated with the development of accessory pathways and re-entrant SVT.

Ventricular tachycardia

Ventricular tachycardia (VT) is usually a re-entrant arrhythmia resulting from diseased or scarred myocardium secondary to ischaemic heart disease or non-ischaemic cardiomyopathy. It may also occur in the setting of acute myocardial ischaemia or even in a 'normal heart', where the mechanism may result from automaticity or triggered activity (abnormal 'firing' of a ventricular focus) (Box 11.1). The most common causes are:

- coronary artery disease
- dilated cardiomyopathy
- hypertrophic cardiomyopathy.

Cardiovascular imaging is used to look for underlying causes.

Chest X-ray

Initial investigation providing an assessment of heart size and evidence of heart failure pulmonary congestion,

Coronary angiography

This is used to look for obstructive coronary artery disease to determine whether this is the cause of the arrhythmia. A left ventriculogram may provide further information on myocardial disease such as size, shape, function as well as mid-cavity obliteration or outflow tract obstruction suggestive of hypertrophic cardiomyopathies or RWMAs (Fig. 11.4).

Echocardiography

- LV size, structure, function, regional wall motion, diastolic function.
- LV ejection fraction (with 3D, contrast).
- Septal wall thickness and mass.
- Outflow tract gradient.
- Valvular heart disease.
- Stress echocardiography: stress-induced RWMA, dynamic outflow tract gradient.

Cardiac CT

- Coronary artery calcium score
- CT coronary angiography

MRI

- LV size, structure, and function
- Myocardial scar
- Gadolinium hyper-enhancement

Nuclear cardiology

- Coronary hypoperfusion
- Hibernating myocardium

Ventricular tachycardia with a normal left ventricle

When cardiovascular imaging has demonstrated normal left ventricular function the following diagnoses are possible:
- Brugada syndrome
- bundle branch tachycardia
- long QT syndrome
- RVOT tachycardia
- fascicular tachycardia

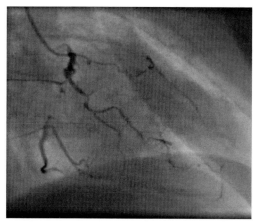

Fig. 11.4 Coronary angiogram of a patient with triple vessel disease and left ventricular dysfunction. The right coronary is intubated and a chronic mid-vessel total occlusion demonstrated. There is collateralization across the lesion and backfilling of the left anterior descending artery (LAD) and circumflex from the right coronary. Calcification is also evident within the proximal LAD.

Ventricular fibrillation

Survivors of ventricular fibrillation (Fig. 11.5) should be carefully imaged for evidence of underlying cardiac disease. This usually includes:
- cardiac catheterization and coronary angiography to exclude obstructive coronary disease
- transthoracic echocardiography to examine for RWMAs and assess LV ejection fraction (often with 3D and/or contrast)
- MUGA may be required for ejection fraction assessment
- Consider dysynchrony studies in patients being considered for device therapy.

Cardiac arrest

Occasionally echocardiography can be useful during cardiac arrest of unknown aetiology to diagnose pericardial tamponade, dilated right heart in massive pulmonary embolism, and vigorous left ventricle in hypo-volaemia.

Arrhythmogenic right ventricular cardiomyopathy (ARVC)

- ARVC is an autosomal dominant disorder caused by progressive fatty infiltration of the right ventricular myocardium resulting in VT of RV origin, worsening RV function, and sudden death.
- Diagnosis: typical ECG changes, usually in tachycardia).
- CMR: RV structure, function, fatty infiltration, fibrosis (late gadolinium enhancement).
- Echocardiography (changes seen late in disease progress): RV function, dilatation, fatty infiltration.

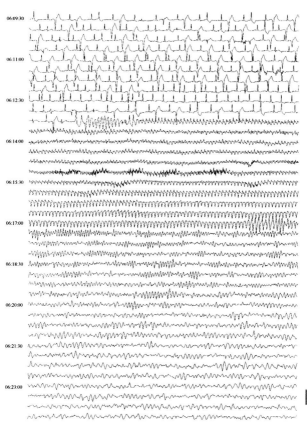

Fig. 11.5 Printout from ambulatory ECG recording demonstrating progression from sinus rhythm with frequent ventricular ectopics to ventricular tachycardia and then degenerating into ventricular fibrillation.

Catheter ablation of arrhythmias

Over the last 20 years the technology for performing electrophysiological studies and catheter ablation has developed such that curative treatment can be offered for many arrhythmias. Imaging was originally by fluoroscopy only, with the guidance for steering catheters being provided predominantly by electrical signals and landmark catheters. Procedures have become more complex, requiring detailed anatomical and electrical delineation, as well as a need to reduce radiation exposure. This is provided by 3D mapping systems, integration of pre-procedural CT or CMR images, and peri-procedural echocardiography.

X-ray fluoroscopy

Catheter ablation procedures were traditionally performed under fluoroscopic guidance which provides high temporal resolution of at least 25 frames/s and allows the whole catheter length to be visualized. However, multiple views are required to gain a 3D appreciation of structures and catheter paths. Soft tissues are also not visible. Radiation dose, especially in prolonged procedures and paediatric cases, can also be a limitation.

3D electro-anatomical mapping systems

3D electro-anatomical mapping systems allow operators to record intracardiac electrical activation relative to anatomical locations in the cardiac chamber of interest. This technology allows accurate determination of arrhythmia origin, generates a 3D definition of cardiac chamber geometry, represents areas of anatomical interest, and maps ablation lesions. This is of particular importance in long complex procedures where radiation exposure must be minimized. It also allows catheter manipulation and positioning without fluoroscopic guidance. The impact of respiration and patient movement on the catheter tip location in relation to the 3D map is minimized by a reference catheter placed on the patient's back.

Several mapping systems are available including CARTO (Biosense Webster, CA, USA) (Fig. 11.6), EnSite NavX® system (St Jude Medical, MN, USA), and the Real-Time Position Management System (Cardiac Pathways, CA, USA). Each system has its strengths and weaknesses. The choice of which system to use depends on the data required, the anticipated arrhythmia, compatibility with catheters, and operator familiarity. When used correctly, these mapping systems enhance procedural success and reduce procedure time and radiation exposure, especially in cases involving complex arrhythmias and unusual cardiac anatomy. The major limitations of 3D mapping systems are that they cannot replicate the true cardiac anatomy exactly, and errors can occur in the anatomical surface that is depicted. This can be overcome by integrating pre-procedural CT or CMR images with the real-time 3D maps.

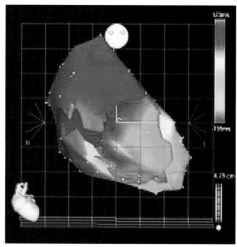

Fig. 11.6 Electrode mapping systems such as CARTO can be used to generate 3D reconstructions of the cardiac chamber being studied, for example the left atrium or ventricle.

Echocardiography
Diagnosis
Echocardiography, both transthoracic and transoesophageal, is important as a diagnostic tool in providing information on cardiac structure and function. It is useful in the diagnosis of diseases that may be substrates for arrhythmia. It also has a role in planning catheter ablation procedures where anatomy is important (e.g. AF ablation).

Peri-procedural
Intracardiac echocardiography (ICE) has largely replaced transoesophageal echocardiography in peri-procedural imaging in invasive electrophysiology as it avoids prolonged oesophageal intubation and risk of aspiration, and is better tolerated.

ICE is useful in guiding the positioning of ablation catheters near specific cardiac structures. It provides clear delineation of the catheter tip on the underlying tissue, which is a critical determinant of procedural success. Many arrhythmias depend on specific underlying anatomy. For example, typical atrial flutter is successfully ablated through identification of the cavotricuspid isthmus, which is an important pathway in sustaining the macro-re-entrant tachycardia. Post-infarct VT typically arises within the border of the infarct. ICE can be used to image the left ventricular scar and thus guide ablation lesions that create bridges from the centre of the scar and across the border to an electrically inert cardiac structure. Such lesions interrupt the VT circuit.

In AF ablation ICE can be used to establish the number, position, and branching patterns of pulmonary veins. It is also critical for positioning both guidance and ablation catheters. For example, the circular Lasso catheter is positioned immediately at the orifice of the pulmonary vein, but has a tendency to move into the vein which, if not observed and adjusted under ICE, can give a false sense of vessel orifice with subsequent ablation too far into the vein. This increases the risk of pulmonary vein stenosis and reduced efficacy of AF ablation.

Where access to the left side of the heart is required, ICE can be used to guide transeptal punctures. This allows direct visualization of the catheter and fossa ovalis, improving the accuracy of the puncture and reducing the risk of damaging nearby structures such as the intrapericardial aorta.

Continuous ICE monitoring of ablation procedures allows potential complications of the procedure to be recognized. ICE can detect microbubble formation, which is a sign of tissue overheating and can lead to clot, char, or crater formation and therefore should prompt termination of ablation to that area. ICE can also show thrombus formation on catheters. Pericardial fluid can also be detected during a procedure under ICE surveillance, and this can be used to guide pericardiocentesis of the fluid. In AF ablation, pulse-wave Doppler imaging can show flow velocity in the pulmonary vein, an increase in which is predictive of subsequent stenosis.

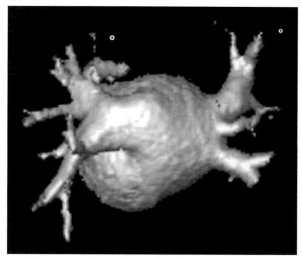

Fig. 11.7 CMR pulmonary venogram. The image is created by collecting a 3D dataset timed to coincide with passage of a bolus of gadolinium contrast from the veins into the left atrium. The dataset then undergoes post-processing to blank out additional vessels, such as the aorta and left ventricle, and leave a volume-rendered 3D image of the pulmonary veins.

Cardiac CT

In AF ablation there are many important extracardiac tissues and organs in close proximity to the areas of interest. Therefore it is now routine to use pre-procedural CT or CMR scans. These give detailed information on the number of pulmonary veins, branching patterns, and the course of the oesophagus relative to the posterior left atrium. This is important in preventing damage to the oesophagus and creating atrio-oesophageal fistulas, as well as guiding ablation. CT or CMR integration is also important in other anatomically based ablation strategies such as non-idiopathic VT and congenital heart disease cases.

CT imaging is performed during a single breath hold, with a simultaneous ECG for retrospective assignation of images to phases of the cardiac cycle. Computerized algorithms are used to superimpose images onto the electro-anatomical maps at the same point in the cardiac cycle.

Cardiac magnetic resonance (Fig. 11.7)

CMR can provide anatomical information similar to CT, without the radiation dose and nephrotoxic contrast agent use. In the future, hybrid X-ray and CMR (XMR) may provide fully CMR-guided ablation procedures. The major limitation to this is that, at present, ablation catheters are not CMR visible or compatible.

Index

Page numbers in *italic* indicate figures and tables.

A

abdominal aortic
  aneurysm 246
acute coronary
  syndromes 144
acute pericarditis 222, *223*
adenosine stress 143
Agatston calcium score 48
Agatston score
  equivalent 48
aliasing 20, 22
Amplatzer catheter 7
Anger camera 56
angina, unstable 144
angiography, see coronary
  angiography
angioplasty 10
annulus of valves 172
aortic aneurysm 246
aortic atherosclerosis 244,
  245
aortic coarctation 256, *257*,
  276, 277
aortic dissection 248–51
aortic regurgitation 177,
  198, *199*
aortic stenosis 194–7
aortic ulcer 244, *249*
aortic valve
  annulus 172
  area 23, 194
  bicuspid 194
  cardiac computed
    tomography *45*
  fibrinous strand *181*
  flow 23
  papillary
    fibroelastoma *181*, *183*
  short axis and long axis
    views *171*
aortic valve view 76, 77
aortic views 88, *89*
aortography 6, 10, *11*, 250
apical window 26, 27
area–length
  method 122, 158
arrhythmias 285–95
  catheter ablation 296–300
arrhythmogenic right
  ventricular
  cardiomyopathy 294
arterial switch 278, 279
atheromatous plaques,
  intravascular
  ultrasound 12, *13*

atherosclerosis, aortic 244,
  245
atrial arrhythmias 288, *289*
atrial fibrillation 288, *289*
atrial flutter 288
atrialseptal defect 263, 267,
  274, *275*
atrial switch 278, 279
atrial tachycardia 288
atrioventricular nodal
  re-entry tachycardia 288
atrioventricular re-entry
  tachycardia 288
attenuation 44

B

BART colour map 22
becquerels 52
Bernoulli formula 23
bicuspid aortic valve 194
bioprosthetic valves *175*,
  186, *187*, 204, *205*
body imaging planes 64

C

calcification
  pericardium 212, 216,
    217, 225, 226
  valves *173*, 174, *175*
calcium deposition 48, 146
cardiac amyloid
  cardiac magnetic
    resonance 134, *135*
  echocardiography 128,
    129
cardiac arrest 294
cardiac arrhythmias 285–95
  catheter ablation 296–300
cardiac catheterization 166,
  167
  congenital heart
    disease 272
cardiac computed
  tomography 40–5
  absence of the
    pericardium 238
  acquisition 44
  acute pericarditis 222
  aortic coarctation 256,
    276, 277
  aortic stenosis 196
  aortic valve *45*
  atrial septal defect 274

attenuation 44
  catheter ablation 300
  congenital heart
    disease 270, *271*
  constrictive
    pericarditis 226
  coronary artery
    disease 146
  equipment 42
  left ventricular
    function 120, *121*
  major aorto-pulmonary
    collateral
    arteries 282, *283*
  myocardium 136
  patent ductus
    arteriosus 282, *283*
  pericardial cysts 236, *237*
  pericardial effusion 232
  pericardial tumours 234
  pericardiotomy 240
  pericardium 216, *217*
  scanner types 42
  tetralogy of Fallot 280
  transposition of the great
    arteries 279
  valve structure 174, *175*
  valvular masses 182
  ventricular septal
    defect 274, *275*
  ventricular
    tachycardia 292
cardiac imaging planes 64
cardiac magnetic
  resonance 34–9
  absence of the
    pericardium 238
  acquisition 38
  acute pericarditis 222,
    223
  aortic aneurysm 246
  aortic coarctation 256,
    257, 276, 277
  aortic dissection 250
  aortic regurgitation 198
  aortic stenosis 196
  atrialseptal defect 274
  cardiac amyloid 134, *135*
  cardiac masses 132
  cardiac tamponade 232,
    233
  catheter
    ablation *297*, 298
  chest pain 148
  congenital heart
    disease 268, 269

cardiac magnetic resonance
(cont.)
constrictive
pericarditis 226
coronary artery
disease 148, 149
dilated
cardiomyopathy 134
equipment 36, 37
gadolinium contrast 36,
38
hypertrophic
cardiomyopathy 132,
133
infiltrative
cardiomyopathies 134
intramural
haematoma 252, 253
iron overload 134
late gadolinium
enhancement 134, 148
left ventricular
function 112, 113
left ventricular
hypertrophy 132
left ventricular non-
compaction 134
mechanical valves 186,
187, 206
mitral regurgitation 192
myocardial infarction 35,
148, 149
myocardial ischaemia 142
myocardial viability 148
myocardium 132–5
pericardial cysts 236
pericardial effusion 219,
232, 233
pericardial tumours 235
pericardiotomy 240
pericardium 218, 219
physics of magnetic
resonance 34
pulmonary valve 202
restrictive
cardiomyopathy 132,
133
right ventricle 162, 163
stress protocol 148
tagging sequences 39, 112
tetralogy of Fallot 280,
281
transposition of the great
arteries 269, 278, 279
tricuspid valve 200
valve function 178
valve lesion severity 184
valve structure 174
valvular masses 182
ventricular septal
defect 274
ventricular
tachycardia 292

cardiac masses 127
cardiac magnetic
resonance 132
echocardiography 128
cardiac PET 50, 62, 118
cardiac segment
models 102, 103
cardiac tamponade 210,
228, 229
cardiac magnetic
resonance 232, 233
echocardiography 230,
231
cardiac volumes 100, 101
Cardiolite™ 52
CARTO 296, 297
catheter ablation 296–300
chest pain
cardiac magnetic
resonance 148
nuclear cardiology 150
chest X-ray 4, 5
absence of the
pericardium 238
acute pericarditis 222
aortic aneurysm 246
aortic coarctation 256
aortic dissection 250, 251
atrial septal defect 263
congenital heart
disease 262, 263
constrictive
pericarditis 224
left ventricular
function 104, 105
pericardial cysts 236
pericardial effusion 212,
213, 230
pericardial tumours 234
pericardiocentesis 240
pericardium 212, 213
transposition of the great
arteries 263
ventricular
tachycardia 292
Chiari network 267
colour flow Doppler
imaging 20, 21, 22
computed tomography
aortic aneurysm 246
aortic dissection 250
intramural
haematoma 252
see also cardiac computed
tomography
congenital heart
disease 259–84
cardiac
catheterization 272
cardiac CT 270, 271
cardiac magnetic
resonance 268, 269
chest X-ray 262, 263

echocardiography 264–7
congenital pericardial
disorders 210, 236–8
constrictive
pericarditis 210, 212,
224–6
continuity equation 23
continuous wave
Doppler 20
contractile reserve 152
contrast agents 126
coronal plane 64, 65
coronary angiography 6–9
aortic coarctation 276
aortic dissection 250
atrial septal defect 274
coronary artery
disease 144–7
coronary catheters 7, 8
fluoroscopic
projections 8, 9
left ventricular
function 122, 123
myocardium 136
non-ST-elevation
myocardial
infarction 144
pericardiocentesis 220,
240
pericardium 220
ST-elevation myocardial
infarction 144
tetralogy of Fallot 280,
281
unstable angina 144
vascular access 8
ventricular septal
defect 274
ventricular
tachycardia 292, 293
see also CT coronary
angiography
coronary artery
anomalies 282
coronary artery
disease 137–52
cardiac CT 146
cardiac magnetic
resonance 148, 149
clinical assessment 138,
139
coronary
angiography 144–7
CT coronary
angiography 146, 147
echocardiography 152
myocardial perfusion
scintigraphy 150
nuclear cardiology 150,
151
coronary calcium
scoring 48, 146
coronary catheters 7, 8

coronary dissection *15*
coronary imaging planes 8, 9, *64*
coronary sinus views 90
CT coronary
  angiography *41, 46, 47, 49*
  coronary artery anomalies 282
  coronary artery disease 146, *147*
  pulmonary arterial hypertension 284
CT pulmonary angiography 284

D

dilated cardiomyopathy 134
dipyridamole stress 143
dobutamine stress 142, 143, 152, 196
Doppler echocardiography *17, 20–3*
  aortic stenosis 194, *197*
  colour flow Doppler 20, *21, 22*
  constrictive pericarditis 224
  continuous wave Doppler 20
  measurements 23
  mitral stenosis *189*
  myocardium 130
  pulsed wave Doppler 20
  tissue Doppler 22
  valve function 178, *179*
  valve lesion severity 184, *185*
dual energy CT 42
dual source CT 42

E

Ebstein's anomaly *291*
echocardiography 16–27; *see also* transoesophageal echocardiography
  A mode *18, 19*
  absence of the pericardium 238
  acute coronary events 152
  acute pericarditis 222
  aortic coarctation 276
  aortic dissection 250
  aortic regurgitation 198, *199*
  aortic stenosis 194–6, *197*
  atrial septal defect 274, *275*

B mode *18, 19*
cardiac amyloid 128, *129*
cardiac arrest 294
cardiac masses 128
cardiac tamponade 230, *231*
catheter ablation 298
congenital heart disease 264–7
constrictive pericarditis 224
coronary artery disease 152
Doppler imaging, *see* Doppler echocardiography
Ebstein's anomaly *291*
hypertrophic cardiomyopathy 128, *129*
image types *18, 19*
infiltrative cardiomyopathies 130
intracardiac 32, 298
left ventricular function 106–11
left ventricular hypertrophy 128
left ventricular non-compaction 130, *131*
M mode *17, 18, 19*
Marfan syndrome *255*
mechanical valves 186, *187*, 206, 207
mitral regurgitation 192, *193*
mitral stenosis *189*, 190, *191*
myocardial contrast echocardiography 142
myocardial infarction 152
myocardial ischaemia 142
myocardial viability 152
myocardium 128–31
pericardial cysts 236, *237*
pericardial effusion *211*, 215, 230, *231*
pericardial tumours 234
pericardiocentesis 240, *241*
pericardium 214, *215*
piezoelectric element 16
prosthetic valves 186, *187*, 206, 207
pulmonary valve 202, *203*
right ventricle 158–61
speckle tracking 24, *25*
strain rate imaging 24, *25*, 160
stress protocol 140, 152, 196
tetralogy of Fallot 280

three-dimensional imaging, *see* three-dimensional echocardiography
transposition of the great arteries 278
tricuspid valve 200, *201*
two-dimensional imaging *18, 19*
ultrasound physics 16
valve function 178, *179*
valve lesion severity 184, *185*
valve structure *173*, 174
valvular masses 182, *183*
ventricular septal defect 265, 274
ventricular tachycardia 292
views (windows) 26, *27*
Eisenmenger's syndrome 284
ejection fraction 100, *101*
electrode mapping systems 296, *297*
electron beam CT 42
EnSite NavX® system 296
equilibrium radionuclide angiography 114
equilibrium radionuclide ventriculography 114
exercise stress 142, 143
exudate pericardial effusion 216, 218, 232

F

first-pass radionuclide angiography 114
five-chamber view 68, *69*
Fontan circulation 278, *279*
four-chamber view 66, *67*

G

gadolinium contrast 36, 38
gated SPECT 116
gemstone detector 42
global left ventricular function 100, *101*
grays 52

H

haemopericardium 216, 228, 232
half-life 52
hibernating myocardium 140, 146
hockey stick appearance 188, *189*
homografts 186
Hounsfield units 44

hypertrophic
 cardiomyopathy
 cardiac magnetic
 resonance 132, *133*
 echocardiography 128,
 129
hypo-enhancement 146,
 147, 148

I

imaging planes 63–95
 aortic valve view 76, *77*
 aortic views 88, *89*
 body imaging planes 64
 cardiac imaging planes 64
 coronary imaging
 planes 8, 9,64
 coronary sinus views 90
 five-chamber view 68, *69*
 four-chamber view 66, *67*
 inferior vena cava
 views 86, *87*
 left ventricular outflow
 tract views 74, *75*
 left ventricular two-
 chamber view 70, *71*
 left ventricular view 80,
 81
 long axis views 64, 66–75
 mitral valve view 78, *79*
 polar view 64, *92, 93*
 pulmonary vein views 90,
 91
 right ventricular inflow
 view 82, *83*
 right ventricular outflow
 view 84, *85*
 right ventricular two-
 chamber view 72, *73*
 short axis views 64, 76–81
 three-chamber view 74,
 75
 three-dimensional
 reconstructions 94, *95*
 two-chamber view 70, *71,
 72, 73*
inferior vena cava views 86,
 87
infiltrative cardiomyopathies
 cardiac magnetic
 resonance 134
 echocardiography 130
intracardiac
 echocardiography 32,
 298
intracoronary thrombus *15*
intramural haematoma 249,
 252, *253*
intravascular ultrasound 12,
 13
iron overload 134
ischaemic cascade 140, *141*

J

Judkins catheter 7

K

Kawasaki's disease 282

L

late gadolinium
 enhancement 134, 148
leaflets 172
left ventricle
 anatomy 98
 volume 100, *101*
left ventricular
 function 97–123
 cardiac CT 120, *121*
 cardiac magnetic
 resonance 112, *113*
 cardiac segment
 grading 102, *103*
 chest X-ray 104, *105*
 coronary
 angiography 122, *123*
 diastolic function 102
 echocardiography 106–11
 global 100, *101*
 positron emission
 tomography 118
 qualitative assessment 100
 radionuclide-
 ventriculography 114,
 115
 regional 102, *103*
 single-photon
 emission computed
 tomography 116, *117*
 systolic function 100
 three-dimensional
 echocardiography 110,
 111
 transoesophageal
 echocardiography 110
 wall motion
 assessment 102
left ventricular hypertrophy
 cardiac magnetic
 resonance 132
 echocardiography 128
left ventricular non-
 compaction
 cardiac magnetic
 resonance 134
 echocardiography 130,
 131
left ventricular outflow tract
 area 23
left ventricular outflow tract
 flow 23, 194
left ventricular outflow tract
 views 74, *75*

left ventricular two-
 chamber view 70, *71*
left ventricular view 80, *81*
left ventriculography 6, 10,
 11, 122, *123*
long axis views 64, 66–75

M

majoraorto-pulmonary
 collateral arteries 282,
 283
Marfan syndrome 254, *255*
masses
 pericardial 210
 valves 180–3
 see also cardiac masses
mechanical valves 186, *187,
 206, 207*
MIBI scan 51
mitral regurgitation 192,
 193
mitral stenosis 33, 179,
 188–91
mitral valve 172, 173, 174
mitral valve view 78, *79*
molecular imaging 126
MUGA scan 51, 60, 114
multi-detector CT 42
myocardial contrast
 echocardiography 142
myocardial infarction
 cardiac magnetic
 resonance *35*, 148,
 149
 coronary angiography 144
 echocardiography 152
 nuclear cardiology 150,
 151
myocardial ischaemia 140–3
myocardial perfusion
 imaging 51
myocardial perfusion
 scintigraphy 50–8
 Anger camera 56
 contraindications 140
 coronary artery
 disease 150
 image acquisition 58
 indications 50
 radiation exposure and
 protection 54
 radiopharmaceutical
 agents 52, *53, 55*
 solid state detector
 camera 56
myocardial viability 140
 cardiac magnetic
 resonance 148
 echocardiography 152
 nuclear cardiology 150
myocardium 125–36
 cardiac CT 136

cardiac magnetic
  resonance 132–5
contrast agents 126
coronary angiography 136
echocardiography 128–31
increased size or
  thickness 127
molecular imaging 126
speckling 128, *129*
Myoview™ 51, 52

N

non-ST-elevation myocardial
  infarction 144
nuclear cardiology 50, 51
  aortic regurgitation 198
  chest pain 150
  coronary artery
    disease 150, *151*
  myocardial infarction 150,
    151
  myocardial perfusion 142
  myocardial viability 150
  pericardium 220
  right ventricle 164
  terminology 51
  ventricular
    tachycardia 292
nuclear perfusion scan 51
Nyquist limit 20

O

oblique sagittal plane 64
oblique sinus 210
optical coherence
  tomography 14, *15*

P

pacing stress 143
palpitation 286
papillary fibroelastoma181,
  183
parasternal window 26, 27
patent ductus
  arteriosus 282, *283*
penetrating aortic
  ulcer 244, *249*
percutaneous coronary
  intervention 10, 144
pericardial cysts 236, *237*
pericardial effusion 210,
  228–32
  cardiac CT 232
  cardiac magnetic
    resonance *219*, 232,
    233
  chest X-ray 212, *213*, 230
  echocardiography211,
    215, 230, *231*

exudates 216, 218, 232
grading 228
transudates 216, 218, *219*,
  232
pericardial fluid 216, 218
pericardial masses 210
pericardial tumours 234–5
pericardiocentesis 220, 240,
  241
pericardiotomy 240
pericarditis
  acute 222, *223*
  constrictive 210, 212,
    224–6
pericardium 209–41
  absence 238
  anatomy 210
  calcification 212, 216,
    217, 225, 226
  cardiac CT 216, *217*
  cardiac magnetic
    resonance 218, *219*
  chest X-ray 212, *213*
  congenital disorders 210,
    236–8
  coronary angiography 220
  cysts 236, *237*
  echocardiography 214,
    215
  fibrous pericardium 210
  haemorrhage 216, 228,
    232
  masses 210
  nuclear cardiology 220
  serous pericardium 210
  thickened 216, *217*, 225
  tumours 234–5
planar imaging 51, 58
plaques, intravascular
  ultrasound 12, *13*
polar view 64, 92, *93*
positron emission
  tomography 50, 62, 118
pressure gradients across
  valves 23
primary percutaneous
  coronary
  intervention 144
prosthetic valves 33, 186,
  187, 204–7
pseudo-severe aortic
  stenosis 196
pulmonary arterial
  hypertension 284
pulmonary valve 202, *203*
pulmonary vein views 90, *91*
pulsed wave Doppler 20

R

radiation effective dose 52
radiation exposure and
  protection 54

radioactive decay 52
radionuclide
  angiography 114
radionuclide cine
  angiography 114
radionuclide-
  ventriculography 51, 60
  alternative names 114
  aortic regurgitation 198
  left ventricular
    function 114, *115*
  right ventricle 164
radiopharmaceutical
  agents 52, *53*, 55
Real-Time Position
  Management
  System 296
real-time 3D
  echocardiography, see
    three-dimensional
    echocardiography
regional left ventricular
  function 102, *103*
regional wall motion
  assessment 102, 160
rescue percutaneous
  coronary
  intervention 144
restrictive cardiomyopathy
  cardiac magnetic
    resonance 132, *133*
  differentiating from
    constrictive
    pericarditis *225*
rheumatic fever 188, 190
rib notching 256
right heart
  catheterization 166,
    167, 272
right parasternal
  window 26, *27*
right ventricle 153–67
  anatomy 154, *155*
  cardiac magnetic
    resonance 162, *163*
  echocardiography 158–61
  function 156
  morphology 154
  myocardial blood
    supply 156
  nuclear cardiology 164
  radionuclide imaging 164
  regional wall motion
    assessment 160
  shape 156
  size 156, *157*, 158
  structure and
    function 156, *157*
  ventricular
    interdependence 156
  wall thickness 160
right ventricular ejection
  fraction 158

right ventricular fractional
    area change 158, *159*
right ventricular inflow
    view 82, *83*
right ventricular outflow
    view 84, *85*
right ventricular two-
    chamber view 72, *73*
rightventriculography 166,
    167

S

sagittal plane 64, *65*
saphenous vein graft *15*
screenwiper study 30, *31*
sestamibi 52
short axis views 64, 76–81
Sieverts 52
Simpson's rule 100, *101*
single-photon emission
    computed tomography
    (SPECT) 51, 58
    gated 116
    left ventricular
        function 116, *117*
    right ventricle 164
solid state detector
    cameras 56
speckle tracking 24, *25*
speckled myocardium 128,
    129
ST-elevation myocardial
    infarction 144
Stanford classification 248,
    249
strain and strain
    rate 24, *25*, 160
stress cardiac magnetic
    resonance 148
stress
    echocardiography 140,
        152, 196
stress protocols 143
stroke volume 100, *101*
subcostal window 26, *27*
supraclavicular window 26
suprasternalwindow 26, *27*
supraventricular
    tachycardia 290
syncope 286

T

technetium-99m 52, 53, *55*
tetralogy of
    Fallot 280, *281*
tetrofosmin 52
thalassaemia 134
thallium-201 52, *53*, *55*
thallium scan 51
three-chamber view 74, *75*

three-dimensional
    echocardiography 17,
        18, 32
    left ventricular
        function 110, *111*
    mitral stenosis *33*
    prosthetic mitral valve *33*
    right ventricle 160
three-dimensional electro-
    anatomical mapping
    systems 296, *297*
three-dimensional
    reconstructions 94, *95*
tissue Doppler imaging 22
transoesophageal
    echocardiography 28–31
    aortic atherosclerosis *245*
    aortic dissection 250, *251*
    aortic regurgitation 198,
        199
    aortic stenosis 194, *197*
    atrialseptal defect *267*, 274
    bioprosthetic valves *205*
    congenital heart
        disease 266, *267*
    left ventricular
        function 110
    mechanical valves 186, *187*
    mitral stenosis 190, *191*
    mitral valve repair
        suitability 192, *193*
    pericardial effusion 230,
        231
    pericardiotomy 240
    pericardium 214
    pulmonary valve 202
    right ventricle 160
    screenwiper study 30, *31*
    valve masses 182, *183*
    ventricular septal
        defect 274
transposition of the great
    arteries *263*, 269, 278–9
transthoracic
    echocardiography, views
    (windows) 26, *27*; *see
    also* echocardiography
transudate pericardial
    effusion 216, 218, *219*,
    232
transverse plane 64, *65*
transverse sinus 210
tricuspid annular plane
    systolic excursion
    (TAPSE) 160, *161*
tricuspid regurgitation 200,
    201
tricuspid stenosis 200
tricuspid valve 200, *201*
tumours
    pericardial 234–5
    valvular 180
    see also cardiac masses

Turner's syndrome 276
two-chamber view 70, *71*,
    72, *73*

U

ultrasound physics 16
unstable angina 144

V

valves 169–207
    annulus 172
    area 23
    calcific *173*, 174, *175*
    cardiac CT 174, *175*, 182
    cardiac magnetic
        resonance 174, 178,
        182, 184
    echocardiography*173*,
        174, 178, 179, 182,
        183, 184, *185*
    function 176–9
    imaging planes 172
    leaflets 172
    masses 180–3
    pressure gradients 23
    prosthetic valves *33*, 186,
        187, 204–7
    severity of lesions 184,
        185
    structure 172–5
    tumours 180
    vegetations 180
variance mapping 22
vasodilator stress 142, *143*
vegetations 180
velocity time integral 194
ventricular fibrillation 294,
    295
ventricular
    interdependence 156
ventricularseptal
    defect *265*, 274, *275*
ventricular
    tachycardia 292–3
ventriculography 6, 10, *11*,
    122, *123*, 166, *167*; *see
    also* radionuclide
    ventriculography

W

wall motion
    assessment 102, 160
Wolffe–Parkinson–White
    abnormality/
    syndrome 290

X

X-ray fluoroscopy 296